'Lothar Gutjahr shows Gestalt therapists, and the rest of us as well, that it is possible to be an intellectual without intellectualizing. He affirms an irreplaceable individual emergent from and within a field without falling either into individualism or into reified atmospheres that engulf the individual. In such a philosophically literate and challenging work, the chapters on resonance are worth the price of the book.'

Donna M. Orange, *PhD, PsyD, philosopher and independent psychoanalyst, Institute for the Psychoanalytic Study of Subjectivity, New York, and New York University Postdoctoral Program*

'Based on the concept that contact is the first reality, Lothar Gutjahr's book vividly describes the inextricableness of the personal and the political. With the development of the author's Gestalt therapeutic field-centred perspective, exploring, experiencing and experimenting become paths to the basic intentionality of psychotherapy: human growth. The socio-political focus on Gestalt therapy is substantiated by an in-depth discussion of person-to-person resonances as field processes. Gutjahr's reflections on the situational field as being real as well as phenomenally perceived are an important contribution to contemporary Gestalt therapy theory and practice.'

Dr. Nancy Amendt-Lyon, *Past President of the Austrian Association for Gestalt Therapy, EAGT member, Associate Editor of Gestalt Review*

'This book is at the cutting edge of the international discussion. It presents and critically discusses virtually all relevant field-, relationship- and dialogue-oriented authors and approaches. Through the framework of a field-centred Gestalt therapy, the author enriches the previous views by dealing in depth with the interpersonal resonance phenomena and emotional contagion arising from contact. His sophisticated, complex, and contextualising approach includes socio-political, economic and philosophical field elements in addition to the therapeutic aspect. A VERY stimulating read!'

Bernd Bocian, *Author of* Fritz Perls in Berlin 1893–1933: Expressionism, Psychoanalysis, Judaism

'The coherence of Gestalt therapy is constantly being reinforced around the foundational axis introduced by Perls and Goodman: contact. But any paradigmatic shift, as this book makes clear, forces us to reconsider many of our concepts that inform our practice, in order to reframe its 'architecture'. For some, this book will be a fundamental approach to this avant-garde therapy, while for others it will be an opportunity to sharpen their skills, since, as Kurt Lewin liked to say: "Nothing is more practical than a good theory".'

Jean-Marie Robine, *PsyD, founder of Institut Français de Gestalt-thérapie and of its publishing department L'Exprimerie, author or editor of 8 books about gestalt therapy, translated in many languages*

'Lothar Gutjahr proposes the necessary shift from the individualistic paradigm of gestalt therapy to a field-centred perspective: "… in a *gestalt therapy of the field,* the emphasis is no longer on *self*-realization of *individual* abilities or of the expression of an *inner* nature. Rather, human fields include strong forces for growth through contact and resonance." (Gutjahr, 95) A highly reflected and fascinating theoretical essay on the core concepts of gestalt therapy, which incorporates the changes in the socioeconomic and political background of the global social field in the uncertain times of "liquid modernity" (Z. Baumann).'

Dr. Albrecht Boeckh, *sociologist, author, practitioner and teacher of both gestalt therapy and supervision*

'Lothar Gutjahr has written an important book which is a serious, methodological approach to understanding and implementing experiential field theoretically grounded Gestalt therapy. Unlike some of the current, faddish attempts at a "New Phenomenology", Lothar approaches this work in a scientific way – not relying on a vague, mystical mythology about the nature of reality. According to Lothar, phenomenology is actually based on real elements, both internally and externally – elements that may be not fully in conscious awareness, but are emergent, and affecting experience, contact, and resonance.'

Alan Cohen, *LCSW, LP, Founding Faculty and Clinical Director at Gestalt Associates for Psychotherapy, NY. As a clinical supervisor he has trained therapists for 45 years*

A Field-Centred Approach to Gestalt Therapy

In Gestalt therapy, sociological, political, and economic research is often neglected or ignored. Drawing on analyses about current societal conditions, this book considers that there is no such thing as a 'postmodern' therapy and offers a new approach to Gestalt therapy.

Gestalt therapy is still currently based on the Cartesian worldview, even if relational approaches are in search for an 'in-between'. The author's approach of Gestalt therapy is based on an idea by the founders: "Contact is the first reality" – so the field coemerges and coexists with individuals' perceptions providing specific conditions, demands, limitations and opportunities. An individual's field is not an afterthought established by the perspective of the first-person-singular (i.e. individuals) but a 'conditio sine qua non'. Gutjahr reflects on both theoretical and practical aspects of the field's many processes of resonance. Putting the field consistently at the centre of his approach, the author describes the main tenets expanding on previous versions of Gestalt therapy.

This important new book is at the cutting edge of the current discussion of relational and field-oriented approaches to Gestalt therapy, and will be of particular interest to practitioners of Gestalt therapy, psychotherapists, phenomenologists, as well as theorists of philosophy, sociology and therapy.

Lothar Gutjahr is a therapist, mediator and business coach working with people on personal and health issues, leadership challenges, conflict resolution, difficult negotiations, project management, and intercultural cooperation. He finished his Gestalt education at the Gestalt Institute Hamburg (GIH) and started his own practice in 2017. He is also an author. www. ProvoCoach.com

The Gestalt Therapy Book Series

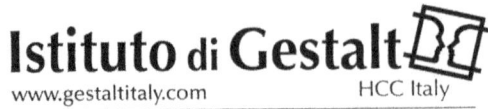

Istituto di Gestalt
www.gestaltitaly.com   HCC Italy

Series Editor **Margherita Spagnuolo Lobb**

The Istituto di Gestalt series of Gestalt therapy books emerges from the ground of a growing interest in theory, research and clinical practice in the Gestalt community. The members of the Scientific and Editorial Boards have been committed for many years to the process of supporting research and publications in our field: through this series we want to offer our colleagues internationally the richness of the current trends in Gestalt therapy theory and practice, underpinned by research. The goal of this series is to develop the original principles in hermeneutic terms: to articulate a relational perspective, namely a phenomenological, aesthetic, field-oriented approach to psychotherapy. It is also intended to help professions and to support a solid development and dialogue of Gestalt therapy with other psychotherapeutic methods.

The series includes original books specifically created for it, as well as translations of volumes originally published in other languages. We hope that our editorial effort will support the growth of the Gestalt therapy community; a dialogue with other modalities and disciplines; and new developments in research, clinics and other fields where Gestalt therapy theory can be applied (e.g., organizations, education, political and social critique and movements).

We would like to dedicate this Gestalt Therapy Book Series to all our mentors and colleagues who have sown fruitful seeds in our minds and hearts.

Titles in the series:

For a full list of titles in this series, please visit www.routledge.com/Gestalt-Therapy/book-series/ GESTHE and www.gestaltitaly.com

A Field-Centred Approach to Gestalt Therapy

Agency and Response-Ability in a Changing World

Lothar Gutjahr

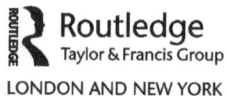

Routledge
Taylor & Francis Group

LONDON AND NEW YORK

Designed cover image: The resonating Field by Marie-Pierre Ficheux

First published 2024
by Routledge
4 Park Square, Milton Park, Abingdon, Oxon OX14 4RN

and by Routledge
605 Third Avenue, New York, NY 10158

Routledge is an imprint of the Taylor & Francis Group, an informa business

British Library Cataloguing-in-Publication Data
A catalogue record for this book is available from the British Library

Library of Congress Cataloguing-in-Publication Data
Names: Gutjahr, Lothar, author.
Title: A field-centred approach to Gestalt therapy : agency and response-ability in a changing world / Lothar Gutjahr.
Description: Abingdon, Oxon ; New York, NY : Routledge, 2024. | Series: Gestalt therapy book series |
Identifiers: LCCN 2023053829 (print) | LCCN 2023053830 (ebook) | ISBN 9781032594620 (hbk) | ISBN 9781032594613 (pbk) | ISBN 9781003454809 (ebk)
Subjects: LCSH: Gestalt therapy.
Classification: LCC RC489.G4 G88 2024 (print) | LCC RC489.G4 (ebook) | DDC 616.89/143--dc23/eng/20231222
LC record available at https://lccn.loc.gov/2023053829
LC ebook record available at https://lccn.loc.gov/2023053830

ISBN: 978-1-032-59462-0 (hbk)
ISBN: 978-1-032-59461-3 (pbk)
ISBN: 978-1-003-45480-9 (ebk)

DOI: 10.4324/9781003454809

Typeset in Times New Roman
by MPS Limited, Dehradun

For Karin, Rahel and Hannah: Your resonances have long helped me to love and grow.

Contents

Foreword

I begin my foreword by quoting Lother Gutjahr's last paragraph:

"Here, now and regarding next steps, I believe gestalt therapy can contribute to a new balance between autonomy and community, as any humanist therapy should. Adopting a field-centred paradigm feels like a necessary next step. We, the practitioners of gestalt therapy should be the first to foster creative experimentation. We should use our own sense of daring, of being unabashedly bold. We need to grow in order to be agents for change in liquid modern times. And we need to focus on the broader field in order to be response-able."

This strong last paragraph might seem un-prepossessing, a paragraph that could we be written by many of us. It is a paragraph that honors the creativity and boldness that is the lineage of our founders, while positioning community on equal footing with autonomy, which is in keeping with many gestalt therapists' increasing attention to ground and to explorations of what we mean by field.

But by the time you arrive at that last paragraph, having journeyed along with Gutjahr, I believe you will have a richer, more layered theoretical and felt sense of what a field-centered paradigm means for therapy. You may not be able to formulate your perspective on a field-centered paradigm with the same intellectual rigor you will find in Gutjahr's chapters, but you will have a felt sense that is at once affirming, liberating, hopeful, and challenging. Challenging in the best sense of the word: challenging us to be our most radical gestalt therapy practitioners.

This book is not meant to be an easy read. It is, however, meant to take you on a very straightforward journey from our theoretical beginnings along the trail of various modifications, adaptations, and changes in the theory. I don't always agree with some of his assertions about what gets left out in prior theorizing, in that sometimes in order to frame his pathway to all that is contained in his final paragraph, some of the nuance and subtlety of earlier theoretical conceptualizations get ignored.

Nonetheless, the occasional biases or over-simplifications are forgivable, in the service of his larger project.

Importantly, there is an important twist, and it is crucial for his project of outlining a profound and consistent field-centered approach. He makes a strong argument about the fact that, much to his dismay, even such a rebellious approach as gestalt therapy has been a servant of some of the most dehumanizing forces of the modernity that birthed psychotherapy as a practice.

He insists that we unpack how psychotherapy theories in general have been shaped by, and pay homage to, some of the most damaging developments in Euro-Western society, politics, philosophy and importantly, rapacious capitalism. He has taken on quite a project, and to his credit the book has a clear structure, a clearly defined argument, and a clear moral position. I sense in his passion, a profound, ethical commitment, which he speaks directly.

He invites us to critique certain gestalt therapy concepts and aims by using the lenses of two sociologist culture critics, Hartmut Rosa and Zygmunt Baumann to radicalize our field theory and our therapeutic practice.

He raises questions about what it means to be human, and also about what kind of humans our theories and practices tend to produce. Gutjahr uses Baumann to describe how, in these times of rapid technological change and the pressures to adapt within an out-of-control capitalist system, the humans of the wealthiest countries, become products; we are measured as 'worthy' human beings by 'performing' our competencies at being human, rather than performing tasks competently. We 'sell' our personalities for public consumption rather than selling our wares or our skills. We 'aim' at individuation and authenticity, rather than finding ourselves as emergent beings-in-relation.

Therapeutic ideas about a process of individuation and authenticity may seem innocent enough, but they have been hijacked by techno-capitalism, so that in order to be acknowledged as a meaningful member of the social world, one must 'show' how individuated and authentic one is. Thus, with the pressures to 'perform' human being well, individuation becomes a task to be managed, not an emergent liberatory process. Gutjahr notes that gestalt therapy, born in part as a reaction against stultifying social and political demands for conformity that characterized solid modernity, carries the shadow of having, in its early days, often pushed practitioners and patients toward a conformity with a very narrow idea of authenticity; authenticity independent of community.

The outgrowth of such pressures to perform human competence, rather than to live one's human emergence, is profound desensitization. As Gutjahr points out, Margherita Spagnuolo-Lobb has been pointing to desensitization for quite some time now, as an urgent crisis of our time. I leave it to Gutjahr to explain this cynical truth further. His explication of Baumann's critique of so-called 'post-modernist' thinking and its damaging effects on what it means to be human will deeply affect the ground you bring into your therapeutic endeavors.

So where, then, does Gutjahr take us? Is there a pathway that can make some cracks in our so-called 'post-modern world', the world of late-stage capitalism and rapid technological changes that can support us and our patients to stay (or become) vitalized? What is the path?

After Gutjahr walks us through Baumann's critical thinking about the structural pressures of what he describes as 'liquid modernity', to help us understand our current situation and its pressures on us to act 'as if' we are individualized and authentic, he then he offers Rosa's thoughts about resonance as a foundational field phenomenon, and how attention to resonance in a particular manner, one well suited for gestalt therapists, provides a chance to 'catch one's breath', to slow down the rushing river that is liquid modernity. Rosa's ideas about resonance might allow us to move and adapt in our therapeutic conversations more adroitly, with a humbler sense of our agency and choice as emergent of field, as well as contributing to, its further development.

For Gutjahr, the path out of desensitization, and the consequent alienation – from our feeling, sensing bodies, from the air in the room, from other feeling, sensing bodies – is resonance. He writes, "If alienation is the problem, then resonance may be a fundamental element of the solution." To this end, Gutjahr describes in great detail, how Rosa and others identify and describe the bio-physical substrate that is resonance. He avers that "resonances, defined as field forces are essential conditions for growth." While resonances are not the same as fields – they exist as a component of field (field force).

For obvious reasons, in that Gutjahr wanted to develop a thorough-going field-centric language and perspective, he hews closely to the abstractions inherent in field theory, and in the bio-physical explorations of resonance. Thus, he points out, for instance, that from a field-centered perspective, when resonance includes anxiety, or alienation or desensitization, vectors and valences of the field tend to narrow affordances, pressuring the field towards restricted adaptive and exploratory possibilities, tending toward stasis. They are part of the first reality of contact. The last sections of his book speak directly to our clinical situation, and for the most part he has worked heroically to do so from a field-centered perspective (I did find that occasionally he put emphasis on the therapist, or the patient, rather on the situation, and that was especially unsettling when he looked at the patient alone).

Staying within the language of a field-centered theory presents some problems in how to speak of the two people in the room. The abstract language of field-centered thinking denudes us of the flesh and blood of making our way together, through sorrow, joy, triumph, and troubles. It sanitizes the struggles I have when my patient and I are suffering through difficult struggles that restrict our capacities. Those times when my patient cannot help me find them, and when I don't want to undergo the change, I must surrender in order to find them. Those times when I must stretch myself into new contacting possibilities that frighten me and restrict my patient.

For instance, Gutjahr writes: "Which field vectors sustain creative behaviour and which induce restricting actions? What divergent vectors are behind our clients' habits?"

Now, I need to translate that question in order to remain embodied. I might ask myself about our emotional entanglements. How are we ensnared, ensnaring each other. What might we be afraid of? And emotions, what emotional processes are flying in, under, around and through us? Because emotions tell us what matters in any given situation. That is, I inevitably need to work to increase my awareness of my bodily sensations, my emotional experience, and I need to experiment with how to dialogue despite our difficulties. And I need to try to sense my patients' experience as best I can and explore with them as best we can. Sometimes patients dispossess me as they require that I stretch and change indoor to meet them in dialogue.

All of what I say here is consistent with a field-centered approach (I hope), in that the explorations I am thrown into reflect an intentionality toward contact in a disrupted field of which I am a part. My point here is that as you read this book, you might want to pause and picture clinical situations so that you can play back and forth between the language of direct experience, and the language of field-centered thinking. It is worth the challenge.

Surrendering to the language of field, reminding oneself to think in terms of a field-centered perspective, helps one to keep attention to various aspects of our shared space, without highlighting the patient as if the patient stands apart from the therapist, as one who needs to be changed. The field-centered orientation expects both people to undergo change, as they find ways to expand the possibilities of the field (including the field of existing-as-humans.)

Lynn Jacobs

Introduction

The personal is political is personal is political

This book is political. How could it not be?! It is about gestalt therapy!

The history of Gestalt therapy has been shaped by historical trends and events. During his early years in pre-war Berlin, Fritz Perls, the founder of Gestalt Therapy, moved in circles where he assimilated a theatrical flair and the ideas of left-wing Freudians (see Bocian, 2010). Like other progressive psychoanalysts, he formed networks with Marxist social scientists, to look beyond the constraints of Freud's original ideas. In 1933 both Fritz and Lore Perls had to flee Germany because of Hitler's 'Machtergreifung' (seizure of power). Political events interfered with their lives forcing them to seek refuge in the Netherlands, South Africa and eventually the US. These experiences informed both their practice and how they formulated their theory of therapy.

Today therapists practice under politically determined conditions which strongly influence and restrict peoples' access to their offers. Regulations of health insurances, and the cost of paying for our services prohibit equal access. Conducting isolated one-on-one therapy sessions in our own practice or being part of medical and psychiatric institutions also influences what, how and if we think about the broader implications of our profession. More often than not, we either need to sell our wares to the affluent or be part of diagnostic processes that institutionalise individuals. Political decisions inform our reactions. Also, societies' structural racism is not something that gestalt therapists are immune to. Often minorities distrust the health system, and the very perception of illness depends on skin colour. It is no wonder that gestalt conferences are populated predominantly by white and affluent middle-class men and women.

Lastly, any therapy is political because our clients are 'political animals' in the Aristotelian sense. The very origin and history of the word politics is closely related to the fact that humans live in communities. Bonds and relations with others are part of who our clients are. Their personal style of relating to others is usually at least one reason why they come to us. Nowadays those real-life relationships are pre-formed by COVID-19, war and ecological disasters amongst other topics. Society and hence individuals

DOI: 10.4324/9781003454809-1

are scarred by social strife, sickness, death, and displacement. If that isn't personal and political!

This book is personal because it is about theory. It is about *my* approach to gestalt theory. Built on many ideas from others, it guides my interaction with clients. Ever since my early adolescence, I have valued science and understanding highly. After a stale and repressive childhood, high school ('Gymnasium') was a breath of fresh air for me. For the first time I was encouraged to think about and discuss politics, social issues, economics, philosophy and more. My teachers valued reasoned dissent. It was vibrant, relevant and a joy. I became aware of how my very existence was both constrained and stimulated by political or social circumstances. Both my parents and grandparents had been traumatised by WWII. My mother became pregnant during the annual regional madness called carnival that mandated sex, alcohol and swaying to loud music. As that was before the invention and mass production of 'the pill', it meant she had to marry my father. Later I could not have gone to university if it had not been for the study grants and loans provided by the federal government in Germany. If that isn't personal *and* political …

In May 2018 I attended the annual conference of the German gestalt organisation (Deutsche Vereinigung für Gestalttherapie – DVG). During the closing event, some members asked participants to contemplate, to really feel the dangers of (nuclear) war, hunger in the 'third world', devastation of the eco-system and more. I was struck by the atmosphere of doom that was being created. Now, only a few years later, these topics need an update. The advent of a pandemic, war in Europe, floods, droughts, wildfires, and more are costing more and more lives while structural racism, sexism, and oppression by fundamentalists of different religions (Christian, Hindu, Islamic, and Jewish) persist. The subversion of democratic institutions by white supremacists and right-wing ideologues continues and the imminent death of liberal democracy is gleefully anticipated. At the same time some people would love to 'go back to normal'. I see that as wishful thinking: "I hate to be the bearer of bad news, but we're not really going back to normal after the COVID-19 pandemic is over" (Polumbo, 2021). Leaving aside the fact that we are not yet *after* the pandemic, I would add: 'Normality' was madness even before the current pandemic. So, what exactly is it that we are hankering after?

As I witnessed during the doom-laden closure of that conference in 2018, focussing on global threats and urging people to immerse themselves in suffering does not induce a sense of agency. High-octane disaster-mongering might be born out of a genuine desire to trigger human resistance, but it hardly activates people. An unhealthy fixation on doom, death and destruction simply makes people more dispirited, despondent, and desolate. Panic is no help when faced with real danger, and depression is not known for its energising properties. So, what can Gestalt therapy offer clients dealing with today's world? What are helpful gestalt insights for change? How could gestalt ideas inform not only my own thinking and practice but perhaps current developments, too?

The first two years of my education as a gestalt therapist were dominated by tiresome discussions foisted upon me by doctrinal proponents of the so-called 'New Phenomenology'. Despite the personal pain this confrontation caused me and my peers, I quickly found out that Schmitz's ruminations about disembodied bodies and seizing atmospheres are not helpful at all. Moreover, grafting those metaphysics onto gestalt therapy would introduce a contaminant of reactionary ideas often indistinguishable from Nazi ideology (cf. Gutjahr, 2018). I also came across esoteric ideas that were (and are) supposed to enlighten gestalt therapy. Some contained genuine spiritual depth. All too often though, they struck me as another form of neo-Biedermeier. As during the era of the early 19th century that goes by that name here is another flight into private idylls hiding from the woes of the world. Of course, the current hunger for spirituality could be considered a rejection of a society in which money is the means of participation in consumption and power. But 'cosmic forces' are not isolated from societal, political, and economic circumstances. Despite the new age industry's best efforts "to exude love, light and purity, it's a profitable one. Economic analysis estimates that self-help alone is worth billions" (Awad, 2021). Largely, the industry perpetuates and aggravates societal maladies although new-age enterprises rather ignore that: There are issues around sustainability because crystals are non-renewable resources. There are issues around labour because most jobs are low-paid, unsafe, and often performed by children. And there are issues around accountability since the industry is unregulated, allowing exploitation to go unchecked (cf. Wiseman, 2019; also Atkin, 2018). Focussing on individual self-improvement, the fondling of semi-precious stones or vaginal 'gooping' in combination with abstinence from politics is very political.

The joint conference of the Association for the Advancement of Gestalt Therapy (AAGT) and the European Association for Gestalt Therapy (EAGT) in Taormina, Italy in September 2016 was entitled "Meeting at the boundary in a desensitized world" (cf. Spagnuolo Lobb et al., 2018). The title itself and the content of numerous workshops raised serious points about gestalt theory. What are the environmental conditions of therapy? As therapists we are accustomed to thinking from an individual perspective. Yet, more and more, I came to conclude that the idea of a self-reflecting individual could (or should) no longer be the centre of our universe. More and more, I felt that theory and practice of gestalt therapy required us to go deeper and come up with more pertinent perspectives "with regard to a theoretical understanding of the subject-subject relationship" (Wulf in Boeckh, 2019, 41). I could and can see no sensible way forward as long as gestalt therapy theory remains stuck in individualism.

My personal turning point occurred when I stumbled on a sentence in (Perls, Hefferline, Goodman [hereafter PHG], 1951/2013, 227; see also

Miller, 2019, 95). I am sure I had read it before, but its radicalism had never really registered: "**contact is the first reality**". Writing about this sentence, Yontef (1993, 272) stated, that in the Gestalt therapy field theory everything is seen through the lens of relating. "In fact, in the lens of our dialogic and field emphasis, the person can't even be defined except in relation to other persons. Relations are inherent and not added on." In that sense contact is the beginning of any encounter. Gestalt therapy is (or should be) about the entire field, not just about one individual treating another nor about the therapeutic relationship alone. Our clients (as well as we ourselves) live in a desensitised world. So, they (and we) are either stuck in a quagmire or together we can explore new pastures. Yet, the proof of any crop is the bearing of fruit. What happens during a therapy session is but one furrow of our clients' fields. Experiences in therapy need to survive the end of a session and be integrated into our clients' life reality. It is my view that gestalt therapy needs to develop a field-centred and therefore also a socio-political outlook or it will cease to be relevant. Basing gestalt therapy on a new paradigm could be an antidote to society's current hyper-individualism, too.

As Goldstein (1934/1995, 385) noted, "unbiased research shows that no empirical data can ever become really intelligible unless grasped from an ideational frame of reference and unless viewed from a conceptual plane". Theory is not an annoying 'afterthought' to practical experience, but a substantive reflection on practice and orientation. It provides the lenses through which we perceive ourselves and our clients. When I started to see contact as the first reality, gestalt therapy became field-*centred*, not merely field-related or field-oriented. As a therapist, I enter the *existential* client-therapist-field and together we *explore* and *experience* heaths, glades, pastures, rocks and swamps. My clients and I *experiment* with elements and forces of the shared field. The goal of it all is not merely a new normality. When contact is seen as the first reality, growth – not treating somebody else's disorders – becomes any field's critical vector and the central aim of therapy. Our clients' skills and yearnings (their intentionality for growth) and our own skills and experiences are as much part of the joint field as are open gestalts and painfully unfinished business.

Based on a field-centred perspective resonance is neither a metaphor nor a moral imperative. Resonance describes real processes triggered by contact. It is a fundamental fact of life and an experience everybody has had. Yet, due to limitations, demands and opportunities experienced in life, the ability can wither. When contact is perceived as dangerous or shameful, empathy becomes a deeply hidden reaction. As in the quote from Shakespeare's Julius Caesar at the beginning of this chapter resonance does not refer to a passive echo or reflection of a contemplating individual (Brutus in this case). It is the self-active response of another I (Cassius). Written at the dawn of modernity, the scene hints at a *communal* outlook rather than an individual-istic one. We only know ourselves because we are known by others! At the beginning of modern times Descartes' said: "I think therefore I am". In today's modern world his dictum, is no longer a useful starting point for cognition or awareness. The 'I' itself is a function or a resultant of being resonated by others. Intellect and psyche are not the raw material of epistemology but a half-finished article. 'You', 'us' and 'I' are concomitant because our understanding of others is necessary for survival, it is physically rooted and felt through the body.

Hence the basic ideas of my personal, social, political, and practical gestalt therapy theory are:

1 contact is the first reality creating the field,
2 (gestalt) therapy should focus on the exploration-experience and experimental modification of the joint field,
3 resonances are physical and experiential field forces,
4 growth is a core intentionality that can only be realised through resonating contact.

The following chapters elaborate on this approach.

In **chapter 1**, I take a closer look at the 'normal' circumstances of our clients who – like everybody else – are formed by societal conditions, demands, limitations and opportunities. I conclude that there is no such thing as *post*modernity, since people continue to experience alienation: from other people, from themselves and increasingly from their own bodies and psyches. "Most people pretend – for themselves as well – that they are happy, because namely, if you are unhappy, then you are, in English you would say, a 'failure'." (Fromm, 1977, 0:11–0:31). So, he concludes people wear a mask of being satisfied, or happy, because otherwise they lose their credit in the marketplace. More than forty years on, this trend encompasses all self-functions. According to the sociologist Baumann, we live in times of 'liquid modernity' in which contacts 'between' humans are pre-shaped by the pressures of exchange value relations. Such reflections are all too rarely articulated or digested by gestalt therapists. I continue to be puzzled by this much like my colleague Parlett (1997, 31): "Given the heritage of gestalt therapy, it is surprising (and disappointing) how subsequent generations of gestalt practitioners have written so little about socio-political questions."

In **chapter 2**, I pursue a question that is fundamental for phenomenologically oriented therapists. How can we understand the unique first-person perspective of another person? In other words, how can we feel what our clients feel? Can we approximate our clients' experiences at all? Is that a merely cognitive or emotional process? How is that different from projections? In my opinion, ideas based on an individualistic paradigm cannot deliver any satisfactory answers to that conundrum even when combined with an interpersonal phenomenology speculating about an 'in-between'.

Answers to these questions remain elusive as long as we base our thinking on the idea of two individuals meeting.

In **chapter 3**, I delve into field theory, considering factors and forces, poles, vectors, and valences. Since contact is the first reality, fields are not just subjective constructs *nor* objective entities facing individuals. In a way they are both. Fields are rooted in reality *and* perception-based phenomena. Contact is neither an inner event of individuals nor any in-between. The field is a whole. Taking the field created by contact lets us avoid the fallacies of individualism and opens a new range of perspectives that can help our therapy practice.

In **Chapter 4**, I consider some situational circumstances of fields. The environmental field is co-constituted by conditions, demands, limitations and opportunities – the id of the situation, as Wollants (2012, 95) called it. In this view, any field is both phenomenally *perceived and real*. It can be explored both phenomenologically and scientifically. The two perspectives constitute complementary approaches; both are relevant for therapy. In this chapter, I also explore the question of how atmospheres fit into a consistent application of field theory.

In **Chapter 5**, I present my understanding of resonance. Inspired by the work of sociologist Hartmut Rosa, I focus on horizontal resonances, i.e. 'between' people. In my understanding, this concept describes self-responsible responses not merely passive reactions. It provides a generical foundation of human response-ability. What is often called empathy 'between' humans is better understood as a field force with specific valences. Thus, it is a meaningful extension of gestalt's core concept of contact and represents the basis of a counter-design to alienation and desensitisation.

Chapter 6 is about the central processes of human contact with the world: our physical and felt body. I consider the German term 'Leib' (usually translated as 'felt body') to be misleading and all too contaminated by ideas of the so-called 'New Phenomenology'. While it is helpful to differentiate between physical processes and what we feel of them, they constitute two modes of the same processes, not separate entities. In this chapter I interlink previous explanations about situational 'Ids', resonances and field processes defining 'intersubjectivity' as the result of emotional contagion.

In **Chapter 7**, I recap the original, 'organismic' or personalistic conception of gestalt therapy. Then I describe the 'relational turn' since the 1980s. By recalibrating the perceptions and perceptive tools of therapists at the time, both approaches provided important improvements of therapy. Unfortunately, both are based on individualism. While many of the ideas and practices pioneered by gestalt therapists so far are still valid and helpful, they need to be transplanted into new soil.

In **Chapter 8**, I bring together the ideas from previous chapters. I describe what some elements of a *gestalt therapy of the field* might look like, how that can solve the issues of intersubjectivity, seize on the idea of resonance and relate to the current societal situation. In my view this approach builds on and exceeds previous outlooks. It allows therapists and clients to adopt the 'middle mode' of response-ability between autonomy and heteronomy.

In **Chapter 9**, I describe growth as the essential intentionality of humans and a natural outcome of contact. Traditionally, therapy is oriented towards treating individual deficits and disorders. By contrast I focus on supporting the field forces of yearning for resonance. It seems to me such a gestalt approach might provide a key to human growth that points beyond the constraints of liquid modern profitability.

Some additional pointers:

• In each chapter you will find several subheadings. They are meant to make my argumentation as clear as possible.
• All quotes that were originally in German were translated by me. Possible mistakes will be my fault alone.
• You will notice that throughout the text I talk about clients, not patients. That way I would like to emphasise an important point. Whatever my clients think about themselves, when they allow me to see them at their most vulnerable, I do not focus on failures or deficiencies. I see a lot of strength, tenacity, tenderness, grace and beauty.

"While there are lots of degrees of freedom for individual organizations and integrations of Gestalt Therapy within the existential base, the field theoretical, phenomenological, and dialogical pillars, much more scrutiny and care must be taken with any paradigmatic shifts which may violate the existential foundation or the three pillars." (Resnick, 2019, 70)

I very much agree with this sentiment. Our tolerance, which stands us in such good stead during therapy sessions cannot apply to esoteric Biedermeiers, conspiracy myths or denials of science as that would violate the pillars of gestalt therapy. It can most certainly not apply to reactionary ideas that blatantly include racist and antisemitic tropes (Schmitz, 1999). To incorporate views of the so-called 'New Phenomenology' is repulsive (cf. Amendt-Lyon, 2018). So, at the risk of sounding like that uptight old Cato of ancient Rome and hoping I have still got my Latin right, I conclude: *Ceterum censeo, novam phenomenologigam esse repudiaturam!*

Acknowledgements

I thank my trainers at the Gestalt Institute Hamburg (GIH) and particularly its director, Marcus Lambrecht. Your openness, encouragement, and resonances have touched me deeply! To my first teaching therapist Andreas Blase, I say, thank you for the music – particularly during those hurtful, conflict-laden times. I am most grateful to my second teaching therapist, Josta Bernstädt, for her patience, support, and challenges to grow … and for kiboshing my well-oiled high-speed train of intellectualism again and again and again. You are right, "deceleration is an essential prerequisite for awareness" (Bernstädt/Hahn, 2010, 52).

I emphatically thank those women of my first training group who were with me during a very difficult time and who socialised my private pain. Also, I sincerely thank my fellow trainees at the GIH. Your resonances are the very reason why I have retained and increased my 'faith' in gestalt therapy.

Chapter 1

Homo homini emptor![1]

Therapy in times of liquid modernity

Apart from systemic therapy, Dreitzel (2004, 75) believes gestalt therapy is "the only psychotherapeutic school that takes serious note of the fact that human beings are social beings". For him and his perspective, this is undoubtedly true. But is it the case for gestalt therapy in general? In my view, therapists all too often limit their attention to the immediate social environment of their clients: their circle of friends, family, and professional surroundings. In gestalt therapy literature, philosophical – especially phenomenological – publications are discussed in detail, while economic, social, or political analyses often remain undigested in the background of therapeutic action. But "in order to understand psychopathological experiences, it is not enough to consider only the individual or the dual relationship as a reference point. A relationship never consists of just two people – there are always other influences at play" (Francesetti et al., 2016, 62).

1.1 Modern times they are a-changin'

At the beginning of modernity, Rousseau stated, "I want to remain what I am" (quoted in Henning, 2015, 40). In 1978, the advertisement for the "tastiest alternative to conventional half-fat margarine" ran as follows: "I want to remain as I am. You may!" (www.du-darfst.de). In my opinion, the background in each case points to serious changes in modernity. Since the 18th century, the everyday lives of people in Europe, the United Kingdom and North America, the social, economic and political conditions there, and the resulting demands on each individual have changed considerably. In industrialised nations, serfs and slaves have become individuals who are now confronted with expectations of having to "present themselves as biographically flexible subjects ready to change in order to succeed professionally or socially" (Becker, 2019, 38). This has a profound impact on psychological structures, behaviours, and relationships. It shapes each stage of contact formation. This trend towards individualisation is not at all a novelty, and it certainly is not a 'post'-modern phenomenon. With reference to Dale Carnegie, the American pioneer of self-improvement and

DOI: 10.4324/9781003454809-2

interpersonal skills, Cain (2011) states that as early as the 1920s there was a "shift from character culture to personality culture". In the workplace, people were supposed to acquire a personality. Later this was called personal branding. As the historical references and embeddings of everyday life were increasingly displaced by more and more anonymous relationships, Carnegie and others believed that individuals could only be successful in economic life and on the labour market if they advertised themselves: "The people who pass us on the street cannot know that we are intelligent and charming unless we look like it" (ibid., 42). As traditional localised lifestyles dissolved and industrial centres grew, personal knowledge of each other dwindled. This trend is ongoing. Individualisation is a phenomenon of Western modernity. Yet it has different forms and phases. Regarding the demands of industrial society on students in the USA, Cain (ibid., 54) states, "These students live in a world where status, income and self-worth depend more than ever on the ability to meet the demands of the culture of personality." Hence, he concludes, the pressure to be entertaining, to sell yourself well, and to never show fear continues to intensify. In plain language, like their ancestors, these students need to offer their physical and mental abilities, skills and knowledge for sale on the labour market. Only now their personality, too, is to be 'improved' or shaped in order to be successful: "The optimisation mania is internalised. These perceived to-do lists swell within us more and more" (Rosa, 2019b, 32). People are expected to increase their own market value by selling their personality as a product. Representatives of so-called positive thinking – which includes large parts of modern management literature and many a corporate trainer – repeatedly claim "that consciousness has direct effects on reality" (Schreiner, 2015/2018, 46). In this respect, success on the labour market (and consequently in life) is supposed to come with the right attitude. Anything goes and individual wishes are supposed to change reality … if you only apply yourselves hard enough.

1.2 Postmodernism is just another (unhelpful) grand narrative

Various publications bemoan a "change in values that has been observed for some time, […] a narcissistic society and culture", and "a general addiction to self-expression" (Becker, 2019, 38). Due to these changes, a large number of philosophers and gestalt therapists have proclaimed a postmodern era. They tend to ignore the fact that this term has been in circulation since 1870, about 100 years before Lyotard (1979/2012) popularised it with his thesis about the 'end of grand narratives'. However, when characterising social developments as an age *after* the end of modernity, clear classifications are usually lacking: What constitutes this *post*modernity? What distinguishes it from the previous age? The political-scientific-artistic answers of those who use the label are as diverse and contradictory as their assessment of different institutions, methods, concepts, and basic assumptions of modernity. Elements of *post*modern thought are said to include:

- rejection of the primacy of reason (ratio) emphasised since the Enlightenment and of the rationality of purpose,
- loss of the autonomous subject as a rationally acting entity,
- new emphasis on aspects of human affectivity and emotionality,
- critical consideration of a universal claim to truth in the field of philosophical and religious views and systems (so-called meta-narratives),
- loss of traditional ties, solidarity, and a general sense of community,
- sectoralisation of social life into a multitude of groups and individuals with conflicting ways of thinking and behaving,
- tolerance, freedom and radical plurality in society, art, and culture.

While the term postmodern implies the end of modernity, what might be beginning remains rather obscure. "At its core, it [the term postmodernism – LG] means the dissolution of enduring, fixed, 'true' and unambiguous structures of meaning, an 'essential indeterminacy and malleable softness of the world'" (Staemmler, 2001, 12). In this view, a multiplicity of perspectives has opened up for individuals: views, needs, feelings, contacts, relationships and goals follow one another in rapid succession, constantly changing and replacing one another, according to changing demands. Simultaneously parallel self-understandings coexist – more or less dissociated – and can be activated or used depending on the situation. If that is to be the brave new world, how can these ideas be told apart from the clinical symptoms of multiple personality disorders as described in ICD-10 F44.81?

Hazy definitions it seems are often the only thing uniting postmodern outlooks. Postmodern political scientists for example express scepticism when it comes to 'objective' truths or realities: "For if what we know of events is discursively mediated, then there is always more than one version of these events" (Diez, 2006, 474). The concept does not become any clearer when Eco, whom postmodernists regularly reference, writes, "One could say that every epoch has its own postmodernism" (quoted in Meier, 2017, 3). Or does the post-modern era represent "one of several varieties of 20th-century modernity" (ibid., 4)? The idea of an end to modernity thus becomes a projection screen for a multitude of possible views and attitudes. Where 'grand narratives' are declared to be over, descriptions degenerate into mere hints of a context. Key words seem to be self-explanatory: "the self of postmodernism [is] naturally related to social, technical and economic developments. Globalisation, networking, deregulation, genetic manipulation, information technology, virtuality – these keywords only briefly hint at what I am thinking of" (Staemmler, 2001, 12). What is he thinking of and how might that be relevant? *How* exactly does the author see the context? The multitude of catchwords exudes a postmodern flair, but it does not provide any understanding of the terminology, their meaning or their effects on clients or therapists.

While representatives of postmodernity are vague on definitions, they ardently pronounce the failure of modernity: "The triumphant march of the Enlightenment has come to an end", they claim and the age of rationality is supposed to be over (Hüther in Storch et al., 2006, 77). In this type of post-truth world, all views are reduced to mere personal constructs. Evidentiary value is no longer established through science but by individual affects. This "primacy of emotional resonance over fact and evidence" (d'Ancona, 2017) establishes subjective, *affective-emotional* evaluations as the ultimate, inescapable evidence of reality. What is true is what an individual feels. Reality exists in the human mind, and nowhere else, Orwell wrote in his novel *1984*. Or in the words of British Prime Minister Blair at the 2004 Labour Party Conference, "I only know what I believe" (Gray, 2017). Where all statements are regarded as mere constructs of opinion, however, scientific knowledge can no longer be distinguished from 'fake news' and 'alternative facts'. In the interest of democratising knowledge, and helped by the onset of information technology, "Lyotard abandoned the noble Enlightenment principle of striving for consensus in reasonable discussion without regret, because the pursuit of consensus always ran the risk of wanting to suppress dissenting opinions" (Meier, 2017, 37). Four decades after Lyotard's publication, these pronouncements seem rather naïve. Today rich individuals, financially powerful corporations, political organisations and state actors use troll farms, cyberbullying and more to manipulate public opinion. The democratic potential of postmodern arbitrariness is as questionable as its demand "not to suppress anything without necessity" (Meier, 2017, 37). *Cui bono*? In a sea of billowing feelings and firmly held views lacking any reliable anchoring in facts, the question of underlying interests becomes blurred: *cogito* something *ergo* it must be so.

"The last few years have indeed taught us a bitter truth. Namely, that interpretations have gained primacy over facts and that the overcoming of objectivity by myth has taken place. But this has not had the emancipatory insights prophesied by scholars" (Maurizio Ferraris cited in Meier, 2017, 131). Possibly it is precisely the arbitrariness of the content of a postmodern discourse that prevents further insights. "Each discourse enables only those insights that suit it" (Meier, 2017, 41). This in turn also applies to the 'grand narrative' that calls itself postmodern discourse. In view of the continuing task to use "the cognitive potentials [...] for a reasonable shaping of living conditions" (Habermas, 1980), the 'project of modernity' is not over yet. The humanistic promise of the Enlightenment is unfulfilled and the methods of clear analysis it has produced are still more successful than metaphysical speculations. I had thought this would be self-evident since Robert Koch disproved speculations about miasmas and soil vapours as the cause of cholera in 1884. His was a fact-based approach.

1.3 We live in liquid modernity

The postmodern emphasis on a supposedly fragmented creation of meaning ignores social developments. It serves as a fashionable accessory for catchphrases that are to signal contemporary relevance. By contrast I find Spagnuolo Lobb's reference to a "sense of liquidity" very helpful (2013, 30f). She refers to the Polish-British sociologist Baumann (2000, 2) who coined the phrase liquid modernity. He saw it as a metaphor, which he clearly distinguished from postmodern discourses, "We remain of course as modern as we were before" (ibid., VIII and 28; also: Baumann, 2012). He could not be clearer; his term describes the *current phase of modernity*. Modernity is not evaporating; it is merely changing its aggregate state, liquefying human relations. The essentially new characteristic of current modernity is the pressure to avoid commitments: "To cut a long story short, if in its 'solid' phase the heart of modernity was to control and fix the future, the prime concern in the 'liquid' phase moved to ensuring the future was not mortgaged" (Baumann, 2000, X). Early modernity dissolved the system of feudalism and state absolutism and replaced them with new 'solid' institutions. Its current form continues this liquefaction, penetrating ever more areas of life and individual living conditions: "Ours is, as a result, an individualised, privatised version of modernity, with the burden of pattern-weaving and responsibility for failure falling primarily on the individual's shoulders" (Baumann, 2000, 7f).

Unfortunately, Baumann's description of early modernity barely touches on non-European contexts and overlooks essential prerequisites of industrialisation: the transatlantic slave trade and the industrialised exploitation of African slave labour. Profits generated by cotton, sugar, rubber, coffee, tea, and cocoa plantations fuelled industrial, commercial, and financial innovations. The wealth generated by African slaves and the riches extracted from colonies had a direct impact on national income and capital investment in the British Isles and elsewhere in Europe. Contrary to older interpretations, slavery was no *precursor* to the Industrial Revolution. The massive appropriation and accumulation of capital jump-started modern entrepreneurship at home (Olusoga, 2016; K. Siddique, 2020). Due to political and economic interests, modernity has always had a dual character: liberation for some and new forms of oppression for others.

1.4 Hyper-individualism is a key element of liquid modernity

Regarding the economic foundations of liquid society, Baumann (2000, 149) states, "The reproduction and growth of capital, profits and dividends and the satisfaction of stakeholders have all become largely independent from the duration of any particular local engagement with labour." Without going into further details here, this seems to be an essential feature of liquid modernity. The globalisation of production and capital accumulation leads to transnational dislocations and (political) conflicts. Markets have been liberalised across national borders and the regulatory power of individual states as well as the influence of organised social groups have dwindled. As part of this development, the paradigm of neoliberalism has become dominant in economies, politics and societies. Unfortunately, this has all too often been ignored or disregarded by proponents of postmodernity. "On the one hand, we can state that in terms of contemporary history we are in the era of neoliberalism" (Müller, 2008, 8), which means that a critique of present thinking, and a critique of ideology is inadequate without a closer look at what neoliberalism entails.

When I speak of neoliberalism here, I do not mean the 'ordoliberalism' of the Freiburg School that has been so popular in Germany since Ludwig Erhard, Minister of Economic Affairs during the 'Wirtschaftswunder' (German for 'economic miracle') after 1945. I refer to the 'Austrian School' (cf. Schreiner, 2015/2018, 10f) and the Anglo-Saxon variant of Milton Friedman and the 'Chicago Boys' that emerged from it. This strand entered mainstream economics and politics through the neoconservative governments of Thatcher in the UK and Reagan in the US. The neoliberal-neoconservative ideas that have prevailed since then are based on those of the economist Friedrich August von Hayek. In his theory he framed reality according to the model of economic competition. For him almost all – if not all – human activity is a form of economic exchange in the market. In such a society modelled on markets, men and women would follow their self-interest and compete for rare goods. So market value determines who and what is valuable (see Metcalf, 2017). This claim is indeed far-reaching. Based on Hayek, the organising principle of society as a whole would be '*homo homini lupus* of Wall Street', i.e. Adam Smith without a second thought (ibid.).

National neoliberal-neoconservative policies had immediate practical consequences – not only in Chile where the radical economic and social policies of the 'Chicago Boys' supported the dictator Pinochet from 1973 onwards. In Germany, too, this type of market fixation has brought about considerable changes in individual living conditions. "Since the 1970s, for example, the wage share has fallen significantly in almost all countries" (Schreiner, 2015/2018, 21), and the incomes of the richest have risen by 19% (ibid., 22). In the meantime, there is enough research to prove the "spread of neoliberal policies since 1980 – and their correlation with weak growth, the ups and downs of boom-bust cycles and, not least, rising inequality" (Metcalf, 2017). Economic demands have eliminated social structures "that stand in the way of the internationality, acceleration and flexibility of capital flows, means of production and processes" (Staemmler, 2001, 13). The economic and social policies of industrialised countries have been based on variations of neoliberal-neoconservative ideas for decades. Thus, it is not a mere 'fighting term' of left-wing critics, as neoconservative protagonists claim. The apologists themselves flesh out the term. "For neoliberals, it is indisputable that without a state, which safeguards individual political, economic and social freedoms, there is no market economy that serves the good of all and thus no 'prosperity for all'" (Straubhaar, 2015). This sounds like classic liberal ideas according to which the state sets the boundaries of markets. Neoliberals regard themselves as 'philanthropists'. Problems such as personal enrichment in their view only exist as excesses in boardrooms. But the extent of regulatory powers they ascribe to markets is revealed by a more recent proposal. Only five years after his neoliberal justification, the economist Straubhaar (2020) proposed the adoption of an *economic* perspective to fight the spread of COVID-19: "Anyone who has exceeded a certain age limit or is particularly endangered to life and limb in case of illness may no longer leave their flat, house, nursing or retirement home unprotected." Everyone else could thus continue to indulge in market activities undisturbed. Ignoring the faulty medical presuppositions regarding the containment of infectious diseases, how is this supposed to be feasible without restrictions or deprivation of liberty? Once again: *Cui bono?* In my opinion, these propositions reveal the underlying focus of neoliberal-neoconservative thinking and action in general. Hyper-market ideologists want to ensure an undisturbed production of surplus value and revenue while minimising damage to capital. What this looks like can be observed for example in the United Kingdom. There, nursing homes have been run by private commercial interests for years: "COVID-19 death tolls at individual care homes are being kept secret by regulators in part to protect providers' commercial interests before a possible second coronavirus surge" (Booth, 2020).

As early as 1997 Bourdieu wrote, "Neoliberalism is in fact a rational religion, rooted, at least in appearance, in a rational view of the world" (quoted in Müller, 2008, 29). Representatives of the postmodern discourse overlook that a new meta-narrative has long since gained currency. Neoliberalism is shaping people's feelings, thoughts and actions, their self-image and identity (cf. Schreiner, 2015/2018, 7). The Italian Marxist Gramsci (1930, §88, 783) wrote: "State = political society and civil society, that is, hegemony armoured with coercion." Hegemony is based both on consent and coercion. In that sense, neoliberal-neoconservative 'truths' form an ideology rooted in dominant economic interests. In turn they bolster political discourses and decisions. In the interests of profit realisation, the current mode of market economy has specific implications for all individuals living in it – including therapists and their clients. Figure formation and contact itself now happen under the hegemony of hyper-individualism.

1.5 The costs of hyper-individualism are privatised

Staemmler (2001, 13) aptly points to the human demands of liquid markets. The labour force is to be as flexible as possible in order to be able to adapt as quickly and smoothly as possible to the constantly changing circumstances and requirements. Taking Descartes' individualism to the extreme, liquefying modernity puts the burden of securing a living on each individual's ability to sell their assets on the market. "The responsibility for the tremendous adaptations that now become necessary is shifted to the individual: the individual themself must react flexibly to changing demands, constantly readjust themself, retrain themself, in order to ensure their profitable usability, their *employability,* through permanent self-transformation and unlimited mobility" (Strasser, 2000). In this hyper-Cartesian isolation, the market appears as the only form of contact between supposedly equal entrepreneurs. Persisting inequalities such as those between capital owners and wage earners or between highly industrialised and rural countries are being disappeared from view. "Risks and contradictions go on being socially produced; it is just the duty and the necessity to cope with them which are being individualised" (Baumann, 2000, 34). These social circumstances inform the conditions, demands, limitations and opportunities of both clients and therapists. Certainly, people in liquid modernity continue to experience traditional coercion by authorities. But the primary pressure arises from the structural violence of 'anonymous' markets. Baumann (2011) describes the symptoms of liquid modernity very appositely: "No one is in control. That is the major source of contemporary fear. [...] We live on quicksand."

In liquid modern times, humans serve the market, not the other way round. "What is actually new about neoliberalism is that it makes the process of shaping human beings into a functional element of the market" (Strasser, 2000). Accordingly, the individual is forced to self-optimise. Neoliberalism is an ideology of the free market in which people 'voluntarily' set themselves up as 'free' actors *and* commodities. This economic affordance and ideological conditioning inscribe a 'habitus' in personalities (cf. Bourdieu, 1982, 227f). What is still defined as an individual psyche now becomes a productive force, individual capital or capital investment (cf. Grubner, 2017, 182, 223, 260). Self is being communalised and commodified while individuals are tasked with optimising their 'human capital' according to the demands of ever-shifting markets. In this view, the postmodern talk about a "tiredness of being oneself" (Ehrenberg, 2004) might describe the fatigue aptly. But without understanding the underlying processes, it remains a vain lament without any momentum towards action.

"To put it in a nutshell, 'individualisation' consists of transforming human 'identity' from a 'given' into a 'task' and charging the actors with the responsibility for performing that task and for the consequences (also the side effects) of their performance" (Baumann, 2000, 31f). In everyday life, people – including our clients – experience the pressures of exploitative conditioning as a call to optimise themselves in view of market opportunities.

- Their *personality-functions* (i.e. their identifications, sense-making processes, attitudes, values and memories) are to be attractive on shifting markets. Knowing that attitudes, values, norms, etc., are socially variable, fragmented and oftentimes contradictory, personal validation can only be reached through success on the market.
- Their *ego-functions* i.e. their mentalisations, beliefs, values, competencies, skills and abilities to appropriate the world are to be optimised in view of their usability on the labour, friendship and love market.
- Their *id-functions*, i.e. their needs, desires, affects, emotions, etc., should be directed towards an 'authentic' attitude in professional life and an equally 'genuine' consumer orientation.

From the beginning an essential – if not the decisive – characteristic of modern capitalist societies has been alienation. Karl Marx distinguished four types of alienation:

- "from one's own product",
- "from one's own activity",
- "of ourselves and our nature", as well as
- "from the other" people. (in Henning, 2015, 111)

The last two points seem to be of particular importance for gestalt therapists. Under the conditions of market economies, processes of alienation necessarily arise; as people encounter each other only as producers, buyers and sellers they become estranged from each other and from themselves. Referring to a process of disembodiment, i.e. an alienation from one's own body, the neurobiologist Gerald Hüther (in Storch et al., 2006, 88) wrote, "Without even noticing it, in the course of this adaptation process, the person concerned moves further and further away from that which had originally shaped his thinking, feeling and acting, when he was still a small child." People do not necessarily become aware of this, but they feel the effects of alienation very well because market demands are embodied. From a gestalt therapy perspective, this is not about the suppression of an original (inner) self, but about conflicts between impulses: "The experiences made after birth in the relationship to other people and anchored in the brain inevitably come into conflict with one's own bodily and sensory experiences accumulated up to that point" (Hüther in Storch et al., 2006, 91). Perls, Hefferline and Goodman referred to something similar: "Almost all persons in our society have lost the proprioception of large areas of their body. The loss was not accidental. It was, when it occurred, the only means of suppressing intolerable conflict" (PHG, 1951/2013, 85). Today this includes the conflicts and contradictions between personal dispositions and possibilities on the one hand, and the conditions, demands, limitations and opportunities of society pre-formed by market needs. This also affects the individuals' psychic representations of said circumstances, their responses and behaviour.

1.6 In liquid modernity self becomes a commodity

When markets are the core principle of human interaction and society the driving factor for liquid alienation from oneself and others, the economic principle of exchange value penetrates all areas of life. Rousseau wrote, "When I sell a good, it becomes for me a completely foreign thing" (in Henning, 2015, 50). The *use value* is related to the properties of an object and its ability to fulfil human needs. The use value of a jacket, for example, consists in protecting against the cold. It is inextricably linked to the material properties of the object: size, material, heaviness, quality of workmanship, etc. But the practical human value embodied in products of work is no longer of (primary) importance in market-based economies. It is the market or *exchange value* of labour and goods that determines a ware's social value. Hence the value of work is not a fixed quantity. It varies depending on shifting economic constellations, i.e. supply and demand. Accordingly, the price does not result from the costs of the production for the supplier alone, but from the subjective assessment of the buyer. The preponderance of exchange value leads to alienation: "If things are no longer valued on the basis of their qualitative properties, but only on the basis of their market value expressed in money, the relationship to these properties is lost, as is the relationship to people" (Henning, 2015, 124). In liquid modernity people themselves, including their id-, I- and personality-functions, are marketable products. They relate to each other accordingly.

The penetration of liquid markets into all parts of society increases alienation as individuals compete with each other in ever more rapidly changing and complex international markets. The "wild chase for social distinction" (Henning, 2015, 41) – in other words, the dressing up of personality-, I- and id-functions as a commodity or 'brand' – are consequences of liquid modernity. They are bolstered by the hegemony of hyper-individualism. Just as in the early 19th century, market conditions force people to offer their labour for sale. Now, however, individual 'providers' are required to offer all their personal 'assets', their entire personality for sale. People's psyche, their character and their whole being turn into a commodity that needs to be supple and ductile. "It is not how I am that matters, but how I should be" (Becker, 2019, 39).

Markets are dominated by owners of capital. Through seemingly anonymous processes, they appropriate work results, dispose of labourers, regulate the manner of executing work activities, steer societal distribution of products and services, and thus directly create affordances for all members of society. This has always been a feature of modernity. While a certain amount of freedom for compensatory "lifestyle consumption" (Henning, 2015, 115) existed in the past, *liquid* modernity has rapidly increased the appropriation and disposal of the *whole* person. "Workers may, indeed they must, integrate their whole person into their professional identity and can therefore hardly escape personal impositions by referring to role boundaries anymore" (ibid., 171). In this context the social philosopher Jaeggi (2016, 12) speaks of a "labour entrepreneur". In the liquid-modern era, every individual is forced to see themselves as a *homo economicus*. Of course, this has considerable personal, behavioural, psychological, and physical consequences. "The market is thus anchored as a reference instance in the individual themself" (Michalitsch, 2006, 94). It impacts therapeutic processes, too. When the product now consists of people's own I-, id- and personality-functions therapy is in danger of becoming just another provider for market-oriented enhancement, even if therapists believe that "today, psychotherapy has no particular political relevance" (Akoun/Heinzmann, 2021, 2). Separating therapy from wider society in this manner, we become alienated from our clients whom we then only see as pathologies or patients. We also become alienated from ourselves, because our own conditions, societal demands, opportunities, and limitations remain unrecognised and alien to us.

"What is new about today's alienation phenomena is that another front has emerged. It is not only the external conditions that overtax the possibilities of the individual and thus trigger tensions; it is increasingly the emotional states themselves that do not fit the subjects" (Henning, 2015, 178). In the 1930s, under the conditions of fixed modernity, Wilhelm Reich (1933/1971) wrote about a muscular character armour resulting from conflicts between an individual's drives and their environment. Liquid modernity penetrates ever more deeply into the emotional and experiential world of individuals. Key phrases of this trend are: creativity and emotion work demanding service to the customer or patient, a duty to be enthusiastic, mental prostitution, alienation from one's own feelings and compulsion to market oneself. Henning (2015, 177) summarizes a "paradox of autonomy" and Schreiner (2019) adds that, in the end, neoliberalism "is concerned with a truncated concept of freedom, namely freedom on the market." When neoliberal or neoconservative apologists appeal to our self-responsibility, it is an expression of this truncation. The same applies to therapists who still only want to strengthen the authenticity and autonomy of their clients. They are unaware that they are supporting social isolation and increasing the pressure on their clients. I don't think therapy should merely assist people to liquify their id-, I-, or personality-functions to increase their exchange value. I agree with Boeckh (2019, 8) when he states, "The often desperate search for the *true self* may correspond to the ideology of an individualised commodity society in which the *true self* becomes a commodity."

1.7 The commodification of I-, id-, and personality-functions aligns people from themselves and others

The individually experienced consequences of the whole person being modelled for market conformity are manifold. Female workers in Indian call centres for example are supposed to "always be friendly and entrepreneurial [and] pretend to be Americans" (Henning, 2015, 206). Their exchange value increases to the extent that they can 'authentically' present themselves as something they are not. The trend is even more nakedly exploitative in online sex services: "Streaming sites [...] allow models to stream live sex shows from their own bedrooms and interact with their viewers in chatroom communities, offering fans an intimate connection with performers of both porn star and virtual girlfriend" (Barrett-Ibarria, 2020). These offerings are no longer just about a more or less credible *physical* performance of sexual acts and ecstasy. Now the market demands a wholesale staging of behaviours, attitudes, *and affects* that serve (predominantly male) projections of desire and desirability. Those directly impact the psyche of (predominantly female) 'performers': "The emotional demands of working as a cam model are much broader than sex [because] webcam performers have to establish connections with clients and grow a fan base, and tap into clients' fantasies all the while protecting their own boundaries" (ibid.). Clients want interaction that feels authentic or genuine to them. Punters as well as purveyors of sexual services (i.e. pimps and owners of online platforms) demand a convincing and authentically presented accessibility that is not limited to outward behaviour. One model wrote, "Camming was taking all my emotional and physical energy, and eventually put strain on all my relationships" (ibid.). Obviously, sex workers have every reason to be tired since they live in a perpetual triple-bind. Sellers are supposed to be joyful or stern, dominant or meek, and forever alluring, just as potential buyers want. Contact is not to be a façade put up in exchange for money but a display of authentic feelings. On pain of reducing their market value, the human products are to exorcise any lingering thoughts or emerging feelings that distract from the task at hand and reduce the exchange value of the experience.

"Authenticity has become something of a commodity now. We are sold authentic-sounding recordings on vinyl records, authentic breakfast cereal, authentic floorboards, and authentic pre-packaged holiday experiences" (Bakewell, 2016). It is no longer enough to *depict* a brand; a person needs to *be* a convincing product. This is as true in call centres as it is in therapy practices. Together with our clients, we are subjected to liquid modern ideologies obliging us to be ourselves completely and align our own needs to the market. We are supposed to 'authentically' feel ever exchangeable affects and emotions. But what happens when fluctuating demands change and suddenly call for I-, id- and personality-functions that a therapist does not have on offer? How can any therapist or anyone else lay out a clearly defined product portfolio that defines their 'core' being as a person without at the same time mortgaging any potential future? If we ignore these fundamental dilemmas of our clients and ourselves, we will promote and foster a severe destabilisation of the ground – theirs and ours.

"The economist and social philosopher Friedrich August von Hayek stated that modern man must always be at home in two worlds. His 'two worlds theorem' states that there is a realm of feeling, of close personal ties, of family and community, in which the rules of reciprocity apply. But then we also must think in abstract, logical contexts and in terms of scales that transcend our private lives. Here the rules of competition and cool cost-benefit calculations apply" (Kaiser, 2016, 1). Only, the differences between the world of work and private life are becoming increasingly blurred, both objectively and subjectively experienced. Leisure behaviour is adapting to the demands of markets, too. Compensatory lifestyle consumption has become big business. What I do in my spare time needs to be planned as it has an impact on the exchange value of my overall 'human capital'. Purchasing things such as electronic devices no longer enriches me, or the time spent with other people. It substitutes contact. Consumer objects, such as films and TV shows, Twitter feeds, Facebook likes, YouTube videos, Instagram messages, etc. lead to additional consumption of prefabricated emotions and affects. What I consume invites me to introject examples of 'successful' personality brands that conform with market demands, while offering projection screens of unlived lives. Consumers watch amateurs 'authentically' acting out roles in what has been scripted to appear as credible real life. They watch 'real' people really bursting into tears of rage, falling in love, having sex, getting married, scolding their children, breaking up or breaking down, patching up relation-ships or disintegrating entertainingly. In this way, consumers often enough compensate for the lack of meaningful contact in their own lives. At the same time, they see behavioural markers for market success.

Medially portrayed narcissism and self-aggrandizement suggest chances of success based on individual flexibility and scripted authenticity. Voyeuristic TV formats such as *Big Brother*, Poo Idol, I'm a Celebrity … *Germany's Next Top Model, The Farmer Wants a Wife, Bachelor/Bachlorette, Married at First Sight, The Spouse House, Love Island, Paradise Hotel, Temptation Island, Love After Lockup*, etc., serve the need to experience seemingly authentic feelings (cf. Stark, 2014, 165ff). They also portray appropriate market behaviour. That is even more blatant in programmes such as *Naked Attraction*. While it is being advertised as "dating up close and personal", that is precisely what it is not. Instead, contacting otherness is reduced to market processes based on crude appraisals of sexual exchange value. Viewers are to ask themselves: Does a seller's body invite consumption? The appraisal begins with a person's intimate zones, which is the only part initially visible to potential 'buyers'. The format suggests that this form of encounter is a completely normal process, such as one's behaviour on a weekly market:

look, don't touch – and buy a pound of flesh! Another show called *Sex Box* focusses on the consummation of the sexual act plus a subsequent baring of souls by 'authentic' performers.

Alongside casting shows, reality shows, soap operas, social networks and lifestyle advertising, there is further evidence of a liquid-modern commodification of individuality:

- *Consumer behaviour as market positioning*: "As early as the 1970s, the French sociologist Pierre Bourdieu pointed out that consumption primarily also serves to denote differences from other people" (Schreiner, 2015/2018, 96). When it comes to consumption, it is most important to pay attention to the relevant individual market; consumed products (including coaching, counselling, therapy, etc.) represent a competitive advantage, as they constantly signal aspirations and attitudes to change that, in turn, increase an individual's exchange value.
- *Psychological dressing up*: A flood of management advice based on "psycho-technologies" (Grubner, 2017, 169f) helps with self-presentation that conforms to market needs. Self-help is a multibillion-dollar business because sellers need to improve themselves constantly in order to remain marketable.
- *Physical dressing up*: Physical enhancements by means of surgery, tattooing, accessorizing, or sport increase the individual exchange value, because "attractive women and men [are] significantly less likely to be unemployed. Moreover, they earn significantly more on average than unattractive colleagues" (*Süddeutsche Zeitung*, 20th December 2011).
- *Emotional conditioning*: Pervasive ads extol the idea that finding love is to be determined by market forces, too. Online dating services such as Elite Partner or Parship, but also apps like Lovoo or Tinder are increasingly conquering the online dating market. Emotions and their physically experienced forms of expression represent a product, as Stark (2014, 124ff) impressively shows. Narcissism becomes a commodity with increasing market value.

At the same time, there are services on offer to compensate for the lack of real human contact. In the so-called "touch industry" (Cocozza, 2018), workshops, parties, and one-on-one sessions with professional cuddlers can be booked. At a retailer in Portland, Oregon, for example, customers can make personal choices based on menus. In Japan, a tranquillity chair seems to be popular because it gently hugs its users. Even before social distancing due to COVID-19, proximity had become a scarce commodity – every minute or part thereof is charged for. Human care workers and nurses compete with humanoid robots that can simulate feelings in a nature-identical way (Sönnichsen, 2020). Although the German Ethics Council says, this should not serve to "compensate for staff shortages in care" (ibid.), here too the law of supply, demand, and profit maximisation rules.

1.8 Hyper-individualism is an introject that destabilises the self

Liquid modernity and the exchange-value principle penetrating all areas of life necessarily also shape the phenomenologically explorable first-person-singular perspective of our clients. "The core of this subjectivity is self-fixation as a commodity. [...] No shred of life is allowed to escape exploitability" (Brieler, 2005). Since the personal efforts of readjustment are only validated (or devalued) with the act of purchase, the result is a "fear without an anchor and desperately seeking one. Living under liquid modern conditions can be compared to walking in a minefield" (Baumann, 2000, XIV; see also Spagnuolo Lobb, 2018, 54). Nothing can be taken for granted anymore and nothing is permanent. There is a constant fear of not being dressed up according to current market needs, not being flexible enough. Where the self becomes a product, the means of production are subject to an expiration date. Market expectations and fashions change quickly. As early as the 1950s, Lewin described the consequences of such a volatile environmental field: "If one is in an unstructured environment, this leads to uncertainty of behaviour, because it is not clear whether certain actions lead to the goal or away from it" (Lewin, 1951/2012, 288). This is what therapists today encounter in their practice rooms.

The authoritarian character and the fruits of the hierarchical and factory society of earlier modern times as well as the introjects associated with that period have been sufficiently discussed (Adorno et al., 1950). The liquid era, however, looks different: "Autonomous alienation is the basic trait of the time" (Brieler, 2005). The costs of permanent social adaptation are being personalised. Hence, hyper-individualism has become the introject promoted by today's hegemonic discourse. "Freedom and autonomy in neoliberalism mean being able to think and act as the market and society expect" (Schreiner, 2019) without being constrained by past decisions, attitudes, values or needs. A liquid personality is a constant work in progress. Its character traits are market conformity, permanent competitiveness, submissiveness to market conditions, an adaptable self, a proactive behavioural disposition, and self-disciplined flexibility. Individuals conduct the corresponding readjustments by and *on themselves* as anticipatory product improvements. "In the course of decades of research and therapeutic practice, however, I have come to the conclusion that economic changes have a great influence not only on our values, but also on our personality." (Verhaeghe, 2014). Of course economic changes afford changing ethical ideas and identities. The challenges of liquid modernity no longer demand rigid fixations on preordained values, beliefs, etc., Moral and ethical flexibility have become market requirements and the only measure of probation for individuals is their sales success.

Since markets are volatile, psychological stability is decreasing – with recognisable consequences:

"The neoliberal character exists as a system of divisions in the subject. It lives in contradiction, exists as an attempt to live the non-integrable: be mobile but take care of family and community; be a team player but think about getting ahead; consume like crazy but provide for old age; distrust the state but obey its laws; despise the old but value traditions; learn the virtues but break the rules; trust the market but accept its unpredictability; plan far-sightedly but always risk everything. Those who obey these categorical imperatives live precariously." (Brieler, 2005)

In this sense, precariousness is everywhere, as Bourdieu suggested (cited in Baumann, 2000, 160). When the principle of supply and demand is ubiquitous, the self becomes amorphous. Moreover, the ground itself is shaky as markets liquefy personality-, I- and id- functions, creating "fragile individuals" (Baumann, 2000, 209). What people once learnt is soon outdated and can no longer be sold, so the person is in danger of being thrown onto the scrap heap. It is a deeply devaluing experience and it is compounded when the individuals themselves believe that this is a personal shortcoming to be ashamed of.

As I said before, the prevalent exchange value orientation tends to liquefy all areas of life and all kinds of contact. This is what we ourselves and our clients experience. We and they are afforded universal flexibility, penetrating all aspects of individual life: work, friendships, love relationships and one's own (cultural) identity, and "modes of presentation of self in public as much as patterns of health and fitness, values worth pursuing as much as ways to pursue them" (Baumann, 2000, 135). Neither work nor leisure nor relationships offer secure foundations on which self-definitions, identities or life projects could be based. Both self-support and mutual succour become commodities, too. "What emerges from the fading social norms is naked, frightened, aggressive ego in search of love and help" (ibid., 37). Existential angst turns into a permanent feature of life i.e. a person's ground. "This is disturbing and in order to avoid feeling it the body must be desensitized. That is why today we have many anxiety disorders (like panic attacks, PTSD, etc.), difficulty in forming bonds, pathologies of the virtual world, bodily desensitization" (Spagnuolo Lobb, 2013, 32). Under the dictates of a ubiquitous exchange value orientation, the entire personality needs to be unsteady. So, gestalt formation is shallow a) for fear of being someone or believing something that is not sellable and b) because market conditions are contradictory. The self that remains is ever more fearful.

1.9 Based on (hyper-)individualism gestalt therapy would be another repair shop of liquid modernity

The "postmodern *amour de soi*" (Baumann, 2000, 66) – here he uses this term by way of exception and without further explanation – is *the* requirement of liquid modernity par excellence. But instead of pathologizing narcissism in individualistic terms or bemoaning the spreading behaviour as a sign of the prevailing 'Zeitgeist', egocentric behaviour is a rather functional creative adjustment to modern liquid conditions and affordances. Extreme ego-centredness is not a disorder, but a requirement of the environmental field. "Competition for the interest, attention and approval of other people" (Schreiner, 2015/2018, 93) is considered normal behaviour in the modern market. The compulsion to eliminate inappropriate, i.e. unsellable feelings in some so-called 'inner' self leads to increasing rates of illness, not least in the form of depression and burnout. Anxieties of various provenance are also rising across the world (WHO, 2017). Indications show that this trend will accelerate and expand significantly in times of COVID-19 and war. Experts fear a wave of generalised anxiety disorders, depression, and panic attacks. No wonder loneliness, the feeling of being cut off from the world or being at the mercy of ungovernable forces, has become an almost universal experience. The experience of personal and even societal efficacy is rapidly decreasing.

If one wanted to pathologize society's demands, alexithymia is another fundamental 'disease' of liquid modernity. It supplements narcissism with emotional blindness and the inability to adequately perceive one's own affects or emotions or to put them into words. There is also a lack of imagination and functional behaviour (cf. Müller, 2008, 76ff). But for me as a gestalt therapist, problematic actions are not based on Freud's idea of repression. People adapt creatively to the broader insecurities described above. It is not an 'inner emptiness' as Müller suggests or merely being cut off from feelings. It is a creative functional effort to avoid awareness of disturbing feelings in liquid markets and no amount of dressing up is going to eradicate that. Existential anxiety disturbs the ground and threatens to render the self an unsellable item. Thus, contact is necessarily desensitized, further stimulating a sense of alienation in relationships. "Alexithymia thus promises the all-important success in certain occupational groups, and the managerial type is now one of the most important in the neoliberal model of life; but at the same time, one loses all real contact with oneself and with others" (ibid., 83). Those who carry their psyche to market must deaden themselves by any means to fake authenticity convincingly. Yet, here is the crux: Whichever emotions people prefer not to feel, they invariably hit the master switch and thus shut them all down. The subtitle of the 2016 AAGT/EAGT conference in Taormina summed it up: liquid modernity constitutes a 'desensitised' or maybe better a desensitising world (see Spagnuolo Lobb et al., 2018).

Due to a "commercialisation not only of feelings, but even of emotional disorders" (Henning, 2015, 179), the increase in individual states of suffering is also quite in line with markets. "Hypomania and dysphoria, in their typical effects on purchasing behaviour, are of great interest to the manufacturers" of medicines (Liebl, 2001, 120). Unsurprisingly, the 'opioid crisis' exists not only in the USA (DGPPN, 2019). If the responsibility for providing market-conforming feelings, affects attitudes and behaviours is privatised, i.e. shifted to the 'inner' processes of 'labour entrepreneurs', their need for performance-enhancing or anxiety-reducing drugs increases; as does their need for training, coaching and therapy of different stripes. Medical as well as psycho-therapeutic regimes serve to maintain or restore well-being. That is their use value. At the same time, they aim to maintain or increase market-oriented performance. They enhance an individual's market value. Thus, they are sought-after products with increasing exchange value. Consequently, thera-pists establish different business models. Some try to measure the success of their approach and make themselves more marketable that way. In Germany, some types of therapies have cornered the market because only they are legally allowed to provide services paid through their clients' health insur-ance. All other forms of therapy thus become more expensive. In liquid modernity real people suffer really. If therapists continue to see only a singular individual in front of them, they miss relevant aspects of their clients' suffering.

During *stable modernity*, F. Perls wrote, "The ego becomes pathological if its identifications are permanent instead of functioning according to the requirements of different situations and disappearing with the restoration of the organismic balance" (F. Perls, 1947/1969, 141). For him, the development of character and personality was the result of processes, such as introjection, retroflection, etc. At the time, he saw individuals reacting to restrictive social pressures. Real freedom did not need character traits, he believed (cf. PHG, 1951/2013, 427). Hence we often see theory and practice of gestalt therapy as being "about the self as if it had no stable characteristics and no pattern" (Bernstädt/Hahn, 2010, 282). Is that still appropriate and helpful when liquid markets urge our clients not to mortgage anything and to shape their future with maximum flexibility? Or is such an accentuation perhaps outdated, supporting neoliberal-neoconservative hegemony? Turning the cornerstones of early gestalt therapy into a support act for neoliberalism would render our founders' ideas unrecognisable. Yet, reciting them as an ossified Gospel of St Perls also perverts their ideas.

I am sure, most gestalt therapists have no intention to participate in any market-oriented conditioning of individuals. Fritz Perls himself did not aim for a 'flexible' multiplicity or even arbitrariness of changing orientations. "He was concerned with 'the idea of waking up and becoming real (F. Perls, 1974, 156), which for him meant 'existing with what we have, the real full potential, a rich life, deep experiences'" (Staemmler, 2001, 16).

Laura and Fritz Perls, Paul Goodman and others were not concerned with more market flexibility, but with shaping life in a self-determined manner, fulfilling an individual's needs. They meant to strengthen self-determination vis-à-vis social pressures to conform, and the gestalt therapeutic process was to help individuals detach themselves from constraints and introjects and come to their senses. For Fritz Perls, "'authenticity' was almost an absolute value and formed the counter concept to the changing 'roles' that people can 'play' and which he valued more or less negatively" (ibid., 16).[2] From today's perspective, however, accentuating freedom, autonomy and self-determination seems outdated and wrong. Social conditions have changed since the 1950s and 1960s. Today it is no longer about liberation from 'vertical' oppression. Of course, many clients still face pressure from strongly normative environments. They need to stop avoiding their own actual desires or needs. But in therapies we encounter 'horizontally' fragmented and frightened individuals, too, who are confronted with confusing and contradictory demands and therefore need support and containment (cf. Gecele, 2019, 320). It is a basic human need to create and maintain bonds. That much is evident from the existence of societies. Under the conditions of liquid modernity, the question still is: *HOW*? How can the human need for contact be felt, expressed, and lived when market survival urges individual commodification, alienation, and desensitised contact?

The "human organism is a socialised organism, and the forms of socialisation are an expression of the respective relations of production" (Dreitzel, 2007, 38). I believe that modern gestalt therapy, which propagates 'true authenticity' does not support the growth of our clients but enforces social relations of suffering. Based on a broader view of the 'environment field', the goal of (gestalt) therapy can no longer lie in liberating single individuals, but in a co-created self-determination that is rooted in our clients' real environmental relationships. "Full identification with yourself can take place if you are willing to take full responsibility – response-ability – for yourself, for your actions, feelings, thoughts; and if you stop mixing up responsibility with obligations" (F. Perls, 1973, 30). Today communal agency needs a higher priority. I am not concerned with abstract humanistic or morally charged obligations to others, but with positioning oneself between the poles of autonomy and connectedness, where real contact can happen. The existentialists of the 1940s, 1950s and 1960s knew that holistic self-responsibility also involves a commitment to other people. "They drew from that the idea that being free is being responsible, and being responsible is being committed, being engaged" (Bakewell cited in Pengelly, 2016). This idea has become more explosive under the conditions of liquid modernity. Alienation is a main cause for contact interruptions, neurotic contact styles and obstructive contact modulations. It is due to the massive societal pressure for desensitised contact patterns. Thus, it should be a core concern of gestalt therapists.

Notes

1   *"Human is buyer to human." Adapted from the Latin quote "homo homini lupus" by the Roman poet Titus Maccius Plautus, popularised by Thomas Hobbes, who used this quote to describe the hostile and anarchic character of human nature.*
2   *See also F. Perls, 1947/1969, 157 and also 1969/1992a, 50, 70, 76, 112, 163.*

Chapter 2

How to shrink a bat

Individualism, intersubjectivity
and the 'in-between'

Many years ago, I read and consequently admired the verve and chutzpah of the so-called gestalt prayer:

> "I do my thing, and you do your thing.
> I am not in this world to live up to your expectations
> And you are not in this world to live up to mine.
> You are you and I am I,
> And if by chance we find each other, it's beautiful.
> If not, it can't be helped." (F. Perls, 1969/1992a, 24)

While the existentialist attitude expressed therein spoke to my personal experience, I later came to realise that it is based on hyper-individualism. Fritz Perls had a "fixed relational gestalt of hyper-autonomy in which empathy itself is seen with distrust and is conflated with confluence" (Cole, 2019, 160). This unintentionally supports market conformity. When conforming with the demands of liquid modernity we "only meet each other when it is mutually beneficial. [...] This is the behaviour of buyers and sellers in a market. If the price and the goods are right, they will agree to make a deal" (Boeckh, 2019, 61). If increasing fears, alexithymia, narcissism, depression, and more are consequences of liquid individualism, how can gestalt therapists still advocate more of the same? Is self-determination, this 'doing my thing' still a suitable orientation for therapists today? Do we have to say farewell to existentialist notions of self-determination? It all depends on how we conceptualise what happens 'between' individuals.

2.1 The qualia problem is individualism's impasse

Starting from Descartes' dictum in the early 17th century ('*Cogito ergo sum*'), the division of mind and body created the idea of monadic egos. This trait runs through the history of modern occidental thinking. When Freud, Jung, Reich, Perls and many others set out to liberate the individual from society's demands and introjects, individualism was the underlying paradigm in

DOI: 10.4324/9781003454809-3

Kuhn's sense (1973). Yet even then, self-definition was not conceivable without taking societal power relations into account. Grubner (2017, 136f) rightly points out that the economic and social upheavals of emerging capitalism "evoked a long-lasting process of individualisation" and produced the modern notions of psyche in the first place. Both *how* we imagine psyche and *that* we imagine it as an 'inner' process, are social constructs not descriptions of facts. With the emergence of modernity, the 'I' has come to be understood as a self-contained, indissoluble, primordial nucleolus that constructs reality for itself and within itself, thus creating personal meaning. Based on this monadic view the American philosopher Nagel (1974, 440) claimed: "We cannot understand 'strangers' or bats because we have a different nature." Because bats have such fundamentally different biological functions and modes of perception from humans, we can never understand the cognitive processes of those animals, he claimed. We can study their physical capabilities and processes, but we cannot comprehend the content of their meaning-making, even if bats were able to report them to us. Nagel thus pointed to the so-called qualia problem. 'Qualia' usually refers to the *subjective experiential content of mental states*, which by their very nature seem to preclude any *intersubjective communication*. That is not a new problem. Hume stated a similar idea in 1739: "We cannot form to ourselves a just idea of the taste of a pineapple, without having actually tasted it." Despite discoveries and the increase of knowledge since then, Nagel and others claim, we can never know what a pineapple tastes like to someone else. Our knowledge of 'objective' physical processes is of little use in understanding subjective impressions and experiences. According to the phenomenological dictum, no one can ever feel what another person feels. However, if that was the final word on the matter the phenomenological gestalt approach would be doomed.

"Self is that conscious thinking thing (whatever substance made up of whether spiritual or material, simple or compounded, it matters not), which is sensible, or conscious of pleasure and pain, capable of happiness or misery, and so is concerned for its self, as far as that consciousness extends" (Locke, 1690/1997, 307). On that early modern individualist basis: How does a 'you' get into an 'I'? Philosophical as well as gestalt-therapeutic phenomenologists seem to have accepted that there is a fundamental dilemma between their own claim to empathise with clients and the inescapable alienness of their first-person-singular perspective. "The uniqueness of the person also presents the problematic that since he/she is unique and singular, *no one* will be able to either *prereflectively* or *totally* comprehend this person's unique experience" (Hycner/Jacobs, 1995, 120). As phenomenologists, gestalt therapists have long assumed that the "subject can realise his selfness only through being a body and entering the world as a body" (Wollants, 2012, 74, quoting Merleau-Ponty). Any first-person-singular perspective is constituted by and anchored in the body. We do not only *have* a body, but we *are* a particular body. No human being can put themselves into someone else's body and into another person's perspective. We can neither give up our own I-perspective nor take on the subjective experience of another person. This dilemma is by no means a merely philosophical one. It is an unresolved conundrum of any phenomenological therapy both in theory and in practice. It renders the whole point of therapy – to feel with someone – unexplainable and unattainable. Yet, the question remains: "You come near me and you know that something is going on. How do you know?" (Wheeler in Bernstädt/ Hahn, 2010, 288). If we assume that we can never adopt our clients' individual, physically grounded, first-person-singular perspective, we cannot comprehend their mental, emotional, affective, physical, spiritual, psychological, and cognitive ways of experiencing. Based on the current epistemological foundation of philosophical and gestalt therapy phenomenology, the dilemma remains intractable. As long as we follow Descartes, as long as we assume that individual monads are the constitutive elements of reality, our subjective first-person-singular perspective is all we can ever be sure of. In this view, everything I can know about 'reality' are mental constructs or worse: projections (cf. Watzlawik et al., 1969). Our clients remain like bats to us.

2.2 Phenomenological epoché does not solve the dilemma created by the individualistic paradigm

In as much as gestalt therapy is based on occidental individualism, phenomenologists have merely circumvented or managed the problem: "In the gestalt-therapeutic context, to the extent possible, therapists empty themselves of all kinds of constructions about the client. They bracket as far as possible their theories and assumptions" (Wollants, 2012, 96). The phrase 'as far as possible' indicates the implied limitations. It does not explain what is possible. The idea of 'bracketing' goes back to an idea of the philosophical phenomenologist Husserl (1987, 61). He called it epoché. He suggested that we could shelf our own preconceived notions at least temporarily and perceive something as it presents itself. Similarly Fritz Perls (2019, 36) wrote, "The therapist should be open, not clogged up with scientific or moral prejudices". However gestalt practitioners today know "that the idea that a therapist can remain outside of the mutual conscious and unconscious influencing and entanglement is an illusion" (Bocian, 2019, 120). Nobody can simply refrain from perceiving a situation from their own first-person-singular perspective drawing on their own experiences. Hence, we "cannot avoid evaluating and judging" (Bernstädt/ Hahn, 2010, 62). Projections are unavoidable subprocesses of contact (Boeckh, 2019, 37). Pretending to put one's own first-person-singular perspective to one side during therapy is impossible. The idea of epoché is just a workaround avoiding the underlying dilemma.

Unlike early phenomenologists, we nowadays allow for reciprocal influences of people in common situations: "Husserl's theory and method do not take into account the mutual influence and interaction of the observer and the observed. The focus of his method was on seeing and understanding the other as he actually was" (Van de Riet, 2001, 189). Yet, as soon as we observe someone – even more so when we interact with that person – we influence, and alter what is happening. We are part of a joint situation. Thus, our clients are no longer 'perceivable as they are', but only as they appear to us under the conditions of our own influence. So bracketing our presuppositions 'as far as possible' does nothing to clarify how it might be possible to bracket anything at all. In my opinion, the tacit acceptance marks a philosophical impasse in the face of a fundamental predicament. As long as we see ourselves as individual monads, we are unable to take the first-person-singular perspective of our clients and leave out our own. We remain strangers in our clients' world and even if we were completely confluent, we would still only project our own outlook onto them. The reference to client-centred empathy as a process "much like Zen" (Hycner/Jacobs, 1995, 49) only mystifies the process even more, glossing over the inherent contradictions.

To solve the riddle of 'inter'-subjectivity, some refer to the so-called intentionality of the subject. Here they draw on statements by Fritz Perls (1947/1969, 40): "the sphere of interest is the decisive factor in the creation of the subjective reality [...] We may even go so far as to say that the reality which matters is the reality of interests – the internal and not the external reality." Based on an individualistic outlook, F. Perls defined the reference point of gestalt formation: "we do not perceive the whole of our surroundings at the same time. [...] we select objects according to our interests" (ibid., 41). If needs are the driving force of any first-person-singular perspective, humans will always and constantly perceive things only in reference to themselves. Objects only become part of our subjective reality in as much as they are exciting, stimulating, delicious, dangerous, pleasurable, or in any other way relevant to our needs. This concept of intentionality goes back to the philosopher and psychologist Franz Brentano. Through the work of Edmund Husserl, it became a central tenet of phenomenology. Thus, phenomenologists demarcated themselves from 19th-century positivism and materialism. They established the first-person-singular perspective as their decisive epistemological authority. In this view, humans perceive reality only ever in relation to themselves, i.e. as objects that are to hand ('zuhanden'). In that vein, "Sartre speaks of a space structured by relations of use, in which the position and orientation of the individual object is related to a practical subject" (Zahavi, 2007, 60). To illustrate this point Fritz Perls (2019, 44) provides the example of a box changing its meaning, relevance, and function 'for someone' with each changing situation. Originally it was the protective skin for oranges, then held garbage, then books, then doubles as a puppy dog's bed and dollhouse; later it poses a nuisance in the living room, a welcome seating accommodation and finally it is transformed into firewood. This may describe subjects relating to objects according to the latters' situational usability. But the statement seems somewhat narcissistic, when transposed to the encounter of subjects because it implies that nothing and no one exists unless it or they exist *'for me'*. If this were so, people could only ever be each other's objects and the whole phenomenological cosmos would revolve around the projection of incommunicable subjectivity. *Homo homini Microchiroptera* – therapists and clients would indeed be like bats and humans to one another. In today's world this older individualism underpins liquid individualism. Thus it supports alienation and the commodification of people.

2.3 People are not like objects because they are not 'to hand'

"Any object of understanding can be perceived and thought of as a thing. But a subject as such can never be perceived and explored as a thing, because as a subject it cannot at the same time remain a subject and lose its own voice" (Bahktin quoted in Staemmler, 2009, 83). Certainly, people can appear to us as objects of our needs, desires or pleasures, as anchors of our fears, surfaces for projecting prejudices and much more. Yet, the philosophical phenomenologist Zahavi (2007, 81) has rightly pointed to the limitations of this view: "Intentionality is and remains a form of object-consciousness and allows us to encounter the Other only after we have reduced it to something it is precisely not: an object." A person cannot be equated with 'I'-less objects. Unlike an inanimate thing, people are "precisely that which cannot be grasped or categorised" (ibid., 82) i.e. an inalienable subjectivity. Objects are situationally available while subjects retain a first-person-singular perspective. Another human being is unwieldy, acts at their own discretion within the framework of their own perceived possibilities. Others can elude our desires, even if we believe we have firmly integrated them into our personal space structured by relations of use: "For humans, things and living beings may be present [*vorhanden*] or also to hand [*zuhanden*] like tools, while humans themselves are never merely present or to hand" (Wagner, 2019, 104). Otherness is constituted by the other person's first-person-singular perspective. It is part of being a subject and as such it is part of our lived experience.

"The self-givenness of the other is inaccessible to me, but it is precisely this inaccessibility or limit that I can experience: where I encounter another subject, I experience precisely that it can elude me" (Zahavi, 2007, 71). While objects can resist my aspirations only through situational circumstances, a person can avoid, subvert, oppose or reject my machinations actively. Moreover the other is "the one to whom I myself appear as an object" (Sartre quoted in Zahavi, 2007, 82). It is precisely when I experience my own objectivity for another subject that the Other appears to me as a subject-being This process of mutual intentionality marks another essential difference between the perception of inanimate objects and human subjects. Another person cannot only evade my intentions, they can in turn become intrusive themselves. That possibility is always part of any situational experience. Perhaps Fritz Perls (1947/1969, 44) had this in mind when he wrote, "Not only do we select our world, but we may also be selected by other people as objects of their interests." In other words: When two 'I's are in contact, neither can access the other simply like an object, because both experience themselves as subjects and at the same time as a potential object for the other. Using subjects as things 'to hand' is ultimately never possible: "I am helpless to 'force' the other to meet me. I cannot unilaterally [...] bring it about" (Hycner/Jacobs, 1995, 97). I can of course reduce my *perception* of another person to their object qualities. But the attempt to do so paradoxically creates an I–It relationship. The other becomes to hand only by me depriving them of their otherness. People can sometimes *appear* as objects satisfying our needs. Yet, they remain subjects and contact is reduced and severely warped in this way.

"An absolutely necessary development is the specification of the difference between the contribution of a (non-human) environment, which does not react, and that of a (human) environment which reacts to the creativity of the individual equally creatively" (Spagnuolo Lobb, 2013, 89). This means any encounter with Otherness not only contains subject–object relations, but also subject–subject contacts. This generates a fundamentally different quality both in reality and perception. "The fundamental quality of mental states is their 'intentionality', for the mind always refers to, intends and signifies something" (Tschacher in Storch et al., 2006, 26). But the manner of intentionality is necessarily quite different when referring to objects or subjects, even when seen on the basis of an individualistic paradigm. We experience people as Others who a) never lose their capacity to resist our wishes or needs, and b) challenge us to respond. In this respect, intentionality is a central concept of gestalt therapy borrowed from phenomenology (cf. Spagnuolo Lobb, 2013, 44). But what we perceive, how we sense it, and our respective behaviours are varied. It all depends on whether we relate to an object or a subject. Especially under the conditions of liquid modernity, people can strive to degrade other people into objects, human capital, or commodities. Yet, people are still left with their own inescapable first-person-singular perspective and thus a human capacity for intentionality and contact of their own.

As therapists we can choose to see our clients as neurotic patients desperately needing our astute observations from the couch's front end. But in real live we do not and cannot relate to people as objects only. Instead we make contact with other people as "*selves like us*, beings with an inner process like ours, which we *have to make some guess about*, at least, in order to deal with them. That is, in real life we assume an intersubjective perspective" (Wheeler, 2000, 161). Hence we see therapy and any other interhuman contacting as a "process by which we come to know ourselves and others, to apprehend our human existence and that of others" (Hycner/ Jacobs, 1995, 58). The central process of understanding is based on *mutual* contact. Here I am explicitly not referring to a normative definition of contact or intersubjectivity. An "unpurposed proximity" (Matt-Windel, 2017, 50) is certainly not always the first reality of relationships and it often does not reflect phenomenological experience. Because another person is not an object but a subject, contact in my gestalt therapeutic understanding describes *every* encounter between separate beings. Contact necessarily requires an Other, a subject who is not a mere object: "Contact with another person involves entering into dialogue without controlling the other half of the dialogue" (Hycner/Jacobs, 1995, 60).

2.4 Defining contact as a mental process of 'understanding' is inadequate

Alas, even if we assume an individualistic intentionality that aims at a subject-to-subject contact, the dilemma formulated at the beginning of this chapter remains. It does not explain how a person experiences what another person experiences. The classic individualistic notion about putting oneself "into the shoes of" another person (Kohut, 1981b, 01:50–2:10) seems obvious and is in fact impossible. Again the dilemma is related to the paradigmatic view of the problem. While seeing people as monads their contact with the world is often conceived as a *mental* process. So the solution to the method problem posed by the privacy of consciousness relies on a "natural human ability, that of theorizing constantly about the state of mind of others from observations of behaviours, reports of mental states, and counterchecking of their correspondences given one's own comparable experiences" (Damasio, 1999, 83f). Similar ideas persist among gestalt therapists: "The very fact of being able to self-reflect prevents man from being enclosed within his reactions to the environment." (Wollants, 2012, 6). People are generically similar, it is argued. Thus, they can somehow do what phenomenology tells us to be impossible. Goldstein (1934/1995, 25) wrote, "the closer we stand in our relations to a living being, the sooner we may expect to arrive at a correct judgement regarding its essential nature." At least, he surmised, it is easier to avoid gross mistakes in describing the behaviour of humans than of animals. Unlike the aforementioned bats, humans share the same physique with each other. Consequently, we are supposedly able to see things from a different perspective – which is essentially our own (cf. Nagel, 1974, 442). Understanding in this view is a mental process of attribution consisting of "plausible suppositions about the subjective experience of others" (Staemmler, 2009, 38). That way the foundation of therapeutic processes would be "mentalisations" (ibid., 40f) or more precisely projections. Really? We cannot understand another first-person-singular perspective so instead we are to imagine it starting from on our own 'inner' workings?

"We all know joy and sadness ..." (Wheeler, 2000, 290). That's true enough. But the so-called intersubjective process of understanding *between* individuals does not get any more comprehensible that way. If the first-person-singular perspective is exclusive, then understanding otherness due to shared genus seems like wishful thinking or an auxiliary construct that only tinkers with the fundamental conundrum. Without a clear account of the specific processes of perception, it remains a commonplace that we are all human. And that misses the crucial point: Any particular 'you' is and feels in the world precisely not 'as I do'. Our second-person-singular has its very own first-person-singular perspective. This is what individualistic phenomenology claims. Mental projections cannot explain *how* interpersonality is established. Moreover, if therapists could only reflect on their clients' experiences and project their affects they would repeatedly need to withdraw from the here-and-now contact. This might be appropriate for occasional phases when, for example, therapist and client verbalise their experiences. However, in affectively charged existential, experiential, and experimental processes, 'inner' musings would only disrupt the flow. Conceptualising intersubjectivity as some form of mentalisation is quite insufficient for gestalt therapy. Reflective withdrawal inhibits or even prevents contact in the here and now and thus limits both the therapist's perception and communication.

2.5 Defining contact as 'empathic' understanding is also inadequate

When a human relates "to another's world, it is through comparisons with his own world, for example in empathic and antipathic processes" (Wollants, 2012, 11). This also amounts to a merely comparative mental performance based on one's own experiences. Only now it is related to affects and emotions rather than mentalisations and projections. Cognitive insight is replaced by empathy – progress to be sure. Supposedly there is an "irreducible modality of consciousness, a special kind of intentionality – often called empathy, empathising, or simply experiencing others – which enables us to experience the feelings, desires and assumptions of the other more or less directly" (Zahavi, 2007, 71). Again, the phrase 'more or less' points to the as-yet unresolved dilemma. If *inter*subjective contact is based on the notion of two separate individuals becoming to hand for each other, phenomenologists can merely apply kludges. And the dilemma persists.

Additionally, the term empathy is defined quite differently by various authors. It is thus too iridescent and much too imprecise. The meaning of the term is sometimes also exaggerated and discoloured by normative moralizing – not only in popular publications: "Without the feelings of such emotions, people would not have entered into negotiations with the aim of finding solutions to problems facing the group" (Damasio cited in Staemmler, 2009, 12). This nexus is a mere assumption and by no means compelling. Negotiations are possible and necessary even when based on a liquid-modern paradigm of hyper-individualism and transactional interests. In a world ruled by market mechanisms, the art of any deal consists of agreed compensations for diverse needs whenever unilateral enforcement of interests is impossible. Gestalt therapists often refer to Buber's ideas about 'feeling with another' (1922/1979). This is usually understood as a deeper understanding of the other person (cf. Hycner/Jacobs, 1995, 22). It still leaves the question of *how* this process takes place unanswered, though. As long as we rest our case on an individualistic paradigm, the empathic bridging of the 'in-between' remains a mysterious process.

2.6 Some examples for tinkering with the impasse created by the individualistic paradigm

As I have said, when authors claim that "people can put themselves in the place of others and are able to see themselves from the perspective of others" (Baer, 2012, 85), they often fail to describe the concrete process of perception and communication. Certainly, people have a special ability to draw conclusions. However, resorting to notions of either mental acts of analysis or emotional efforts seems inadequate. Both are based on notions of pre-formed monads who *subsequently* encounter an external reality which they then process internally. Based on the individualistic paradigm, it remains a mystery how thoughts and feelings can pass from one organism to another – unless one assumes overarching qualities, such as Schmitz's (1999, 36) 'Einleibung', i.e. incorporation through the felt body. Other authors cite body memory as a crucial factor of inter-subjectivity (Baer, 2012, 72). Yet the substitution of a monadic mind with an equally disconnected felt-body, does not change the one-sidedness of the individualistic paradigm. Although Baer (2012, 74) explains that explicit memory is not the same as body memory, "explicit remembering is embedded in body memory. [...] In this context, body memory is the primary one." This provides a hint at what is happening but only sketches the connection in the broadest of terms. Mental transpositions as well as intercorporeal perceptions postulate the existence of an individual *before* its environment:

- The 'I' is already certain of itself, so that it can relate the respective circumstances to itself and, if necessary, recognise them as relevant (a threat, a treat, etc.).
- The 'I' at this point already has the ability to distinguish between 'I' and 'not-I'. "For a phenomenon to exist and be perceivable, it must stand in contrast to something else, differ from something else, be different" (Friedländer, 2009, 155).
- The 'I' has sensory, motor, biochemical, psychological, or other reactive properties that it can employ in a goal-oriented way.

Petzold (1992, 155), too, fails to explain how we know or feel what others know or feel: "Although everyone else cannot be like me, this familiarity [...] remains with me. I recognise approximately where the client is at the moment." Approximately? As far as possible? As best we can? *How* can we? How far? What is our best here? Presented in this way the process remains vague and Petzold makes do with a metaphor: "On every expedition into a wilderness I encounter unexpected circumstances, something that did not exist there before. But it helps me if I have been there a few times before and the area seems familiar" (ibid.). Sadly he contradicts his own statement regarding interventions: "My head is of no use to me in finding out 'when'. It can only guide by rules and by how something happened a few times before" (ibid., 158). Of course it is true that one's own therapeutic experiences help with recognising what is going on 'in' the other. But this does not solve the fundamental problem of intersubjectivity. It cannot explain the epistemological dilemma between the 'I'-experience of another (e.g. a client) and my experience of that stranger. Petzold's explanations like many others remain stuck in a diffuse 'something like this'.

At first glance Staemmler's idea (2009, 226) seems to be helpful. He proposes to understand human empathy in psychotherapy "as an intersubjective, reciprocal process", which takes place bodily in different ways. But his characterisation of the 'intersubjective' processes is too vague. The adjective suggests processes *between* individuals, what Spagnuolo Lobb (2013, 98) – similar to Francesetti (2020, 47) – calls "the experiential space between the I and the you, or between the internal experience and the environmental influence". Dictionaries define in-between as something third (a thing, a space or the like) between and apart from two other objects (cf. https://dictionary.cambridge. org). Phenomenological references to an in-between are also quite frequent: "The infant's relation to the world can be described [...] as a pure in-between corporeality" (Fuchs, 2000a, 275). This third often references ideas about *intercorporéité* of the French phenomenologist Merleau-Ponty (e.g. Baer, 2012, 61). However, on the basis of an individualist paradigm, the holistic process is fragmented into a trinity: I, Thou and something separate from, yet connected to the individuals. This supposes an "experiential field that is created between patient and therapist" (Donna Orange in Spagnuolo Lobb, 2013, 26). Unfortunately it breaks up the situation into different locales and foams up the in-between into another postmodern narrative. Staemmler (2009, 114) writes about *reciprocal* actions that lead people to feel "in their own bodies what they perceive in the body of the other, because they spontaneously actively comprehend in their own bodies what they have perceived of the bodily events of the other". While he touches on ideas elaborated in chapter 6, it is his view of reciprocity in the context of *mental-emotional empathy*, that keeps him within the confines of a strangely enduring individualism. When seen as a "realm of the imagination, of fantasy, in which I establish references" (Petersen, 2020, 25), the in-between then becomes entirely vague and open to esoteric projections.

2.7 Conclusion: The individualistic paradigm limits the possibilities of gestalt therapy

Fritz Perls (1947/1969, 43) wrote, "Is the organism the primary factor and is the world created by its needs? Or is there primarily a world to which the organism responds? Both views are correct *in toto*." What could be misunderstood as a paradox I still find a helpful orientation, because neither the inside of an individual nor external environments are primary. It is the underlying paradigm i.e. the individualistic conception that reifies an in-between and tears up the perception of holistic situations. Starting from that oh-so-Cartesian basis, the question posed at the beginning about intersubjectivity cannot be answered. Whether mind- or body-based, whether seen as a mental or an emotional process, 'I do my thing' denotes an inescapable first-person-singular perspective that might as well be that of a bat. Subjectivity certainly establishes a specifically human capacity for a) self-determination, b) reaching out to others, and c) resistance to outside impositions. It is a fundamentally different type of contact than an intentionality reaching for functional objects. Based on an individualistic view of the world and of human beings and even more so within the narrow confines of its neoliberal-neoconservative exaggeration, social connectedness is lost from view. Contact becomes a mere afterthought of a pre-defined humanness. Regarding the gestalt prayer quoted above, Joseph Zinker wrote in 1977 (161): "The outlook is not adequate to deal with the notion of social responsibility, of people taking care of each other in group therapy or any other community setting." Based on an individualistic paradigm, it remains inexplicable how human sociality is produced because it misses the essence of subject-to-subject contact. Every person is a subject, each with their own way of experiencing and acting, with specific social references and with their own authority and responsibility. Hence an encounter of first-person-singulars is something fundamentally different from accessing objects. Although the expansion of exchange-value-relations obscures that more and more, otherness is not 'to hand'.

"I am the sole owner of my experiential life. [...] No one makes me do what I do; no one else can be held responsible for my behaviour" (ibid., 84). That is both right and wrong in my view: yes, I am responsible for my behaviour but no, other people can influence me. If we start from an existentialist orientation, accountability implies a co-responsibility for the effects of one's actions (Bernstädt/Hahn, 2010, 111). However, if social stewardship is to be more than a moralistic claim and something different from hyper-individualistic freedom, the question of intersubjectivity requires a *consistent* gestalt therapeutic answer. Contact is both the first reality of human life and a solution to the theoretical paradox mentioned at the beginning. However, this notion can only realise its full potential if it's based on a field-centred approach.

Chapter 3

Contact is a field's first reality

Beginning in early childhood, we gradually come to experience ourselves as individuals: "Having a sense of self is not only required for knowing, in the proper sense, but may influence the processing of whatever gets to be known" (Damasio, 1999, 19). Again and again, during the course of our development, we perceive our physical being in the world as distinct from others. This reaffirms our perspective as separate individuals and constitutes our first-person-singular perspective, i.e. this ineluctable zero point from which we relate to the world. At the same time, we experience the sun setting in the west rather the earth's rotation. That is to say: Factually, individuals are never first 'for themselves' and *then* a component of their environment. When we become aware of our 'surroundings', we have already been in contact with others for a long and formative time. In that sense humans are first-person-plurals from the beginning, both physically because their survival as infants depends on others, and experientially because they are (at least dimly) aware of that dependency. When infants cry for food, they always experience two dimensions simultaneously and holistically: the needs of their own body (separate from other bodies) and the essential necessity for contact with other bodies (and things) in the environment. "We don't have a duality of a need plus a cathected object (in gestalt psychology called *Aufforderungscharakter*, affordance), but a single event" (...F. Perls, 2019, 30). Yet, gestalt therapy has straddled the paradox of both the occidental *'cogito ergo sum'* and field theory. While exaggerating the importance of the individual, gestalt therapists have always insisted: "The definition of an organism is the definition of an organism/environment field" (PHG, 1951/2013, 258). Field concepts have been part of gestalt therapy theory while the underlying paradigm remained an individualistic one. No one ever exists without contact to another human because "every organism lives embedded in an environment with which it exchanges energy, matter and information" (Dreitzel, 2007, 38). The verb indicates the underpinning: discrete entities are seen as being *embedded*. Yet, if contact is the first reality it makes no sense to talk of individuals somehow rooted in their environment. Based on the Cartesian perspective, an individual is an intellectual abstraction rather than a reality, even when the

DOI: 10.4324/9781003454809-4

environment is defined as a central characteristic. As contact is the first reality, any first-person-singular perspective is a function of the field. The first-person-plural is primary.

3.1 Fields are structured by real 'ids' and perceived by a first-person-singular

The notion of fields in physics "appeared from the eighteenth century as a concept to help elucidate 'action at a distance'" (Parlett, 1997, 18). There, the term describes the spatial distribution of a force action that can be exerted on electric charges and currents. Unlike conventional fields these are not defined by spatial proximity, but by forces that relate to each other even if they are not close to one another. Later similar ideas were applied to social sciences. When creating gestalt therapy, Laura and Fritz Perls specifically referred to the field theory of Kurt Lewin. For him fields are characterised by their structure and their processes of change. Taking the term from physics Lewin did not see it as a mere metaphor. Rather he conceived of a dynamic model for analysing individual and social behaviour based on the description of relationships: "The structure of the living space is the spatial relationship of its parts" and forces (Lewin, 1951/2012, 284 and 292f). For him, field structures encompass poles and forces as well as their correlations, processes and changes, i.e. a totality of simultaneously existing facts. "Psychology must regard the habitat, which includes the person and his environment, as a field" (ibid., 226). The poles and forces, their valences, strengths, and directions do not necessarily relate to each other harmoniously, yet they constitute discernible structured processes, i.e. a unified field.

Of course any field also has connections to structures, forces, and processes beyond its own borders. These perimeters both separate and connect 'inside' and 'outside' of a given field. What distinguishes both sides of the 'fence' is relative: "the degree of dependence between any two parts within a natural whole is greater than between any part and a region outside the whole" (ibid., 341). This describes a discernible segue of forces and processes, not a separation between an entity and its surroundings. A field in its entirety is an open system encompassing different processes and 'parts' as well as interaction with other fields. For gestalt therapists it has long been clear that a boundary is not a point of separation nor really the locale of contact, but the *processes of contacting* itself. Based on this view, it makes no sense to talk about monads in an environment and space in between them.

Whatever the specific characteristics of a given field might be, it is the entire habitat that is at the centre of (therapeutic) attention because the behaviour of an individual is the function of the so-called present field, "which is in constant flux and in which different forces (vectors) act on the individual. This dynamic field is not only influenced by the actual present situation" (Frey: Preface in Lewin, 1951/2012, 7). Hopes and fears of the individual regarding their future, as well as views about their own past, play a part. In this context Spagnuolo Lobb (2018, 53) speaks of the experiential ground of the field:

> "Life is made up of events that take place in certain situations, perceived by each of us in a here-and-now, grounded on previous contacts and intended into the future: thoughts; neurobiological, emotional, and behavioural reactions; and climate and social conditions form an indivisible whole: the experiential ground of the field."

That squares with Lewin's ideas (1951/2012, 69). Where Spagnuolo Lobb speaks of now-for-next as a fundamental human intentionality, a consistent field orientation would call it forces and valences of the field. Intentionalities are functions of a field not the expression of a being's essence. In a similar vein, Francesetti (2020, 44) writes about 'phenomenal fields' which for him are phenomena of experience that emerge during an encounter. Since many different forms of experience and limits can arise in this field they might be seen as the horizon *of all possible forms*. "The phenomenal field is generated by everything relevant and extends in space and time as far as it produces a difference in experience – these are its limits." What seems important to me is that the field

a is clearly larger than what can be experienced here-and-now, i.e. larger than a current I–thou contact;
b encompasses the entire ground, thus offering considerably and substantially more than just the figures that emerge at any given moment;
c is not merely thought of or sensed. Fields are not merely phenomenological experiences or figments of imagination. They comprise physical conditions, possibilities, demands and limitations, too. These circumstances are given, handed down and subjectively stumbled on. They constitute real forces and structures, that afford the possibilities Francesetti talks about.
d is a whole not an assortment of its parts.

"The phenomenal field is something that arises between us and around us in the encounter", Francesetti (2020, 44) says. Unfortunately, he builds his view on neo-phenomenological speculations, describing a field existing "as a quasi-thing that is fleetingly present among the participants" (ibid., 45). Such not-really-things might perhaps describe the subjective processes of certain perceptions. But the notions of spacelessly poured-out quasi-things wrongly misrepresent forces as agents having their own volition in the field. That mystifies rather than elucidates what is going on.

Laura and Fritz Perls combined concepts of gestalt psychology with those of fields and forces.

"Lewin starts from the basic assumption that behaviour is goal-oriented, and a function of the 'habitat' given to the individual at a given time. The habitat comprises both the person themselves and their environment; it is divided into individual regions, each of which has a different calling character for the person (valences) and which are delimited from each other by barriers of varying strength. The concrete behaviour (locomotion) can be represented vector-psychologically as a resultant of the attractive and repulsive field forces acting on the individual." (Wenninger, 2000)

This describes the field perspective quite well: What a person does (locomotion) is the result of forces and their valences. Of course those forces can be both physical objects and immaterial notions, ideas or emotions. If however the field is seen only as "surrounding space of an embodied subject in the broadest sense" (Fuchs, 2019b, 117f), the field is reduced to a mere afterthought. Once more the individual is seen as pre-existing and Cartesian individualism prevails. What in reality is a unified field is thus being dissected into different parts facing each other. Still these 'parts' – the individual and its surroundings – are physically grounded, coexistent, and related to each other. Also the field is not seen as a mere cognition. So that is different from classical individualism. However, Fuchs' quote also demonstrates that, for all his holistic verbiage, he still thinks of an individual as an entity in a surrounding space. Figuratively speaking, the human being remains the centre around which everything revolves.

"A question becomes inevitable at some point: is 'the field' ultimately just a metaphor, a useful derivative concept and frame of reference that can be used to explain what is otherwise difficult to explain? Or is 'something there' in the form of an explicit energy field in the 'space between'?" (Parlett, 2005, 60). When the field is not conceptualised as a structured unit this question is bound to appear. On the one hand, I agree with Francesetti (2020, 46) when he states that a field is not just a metaphor for what goes on. Instead, field theory endeavours to describe actual processes. On the other hand, however, I reject any speculations about a metaphysical trinity of I, Thou and in-between. Instead, I focus on the structures and processes of fields, the way the poles relate to each other, the forces and valences that are present, and the boundary processes describing contact with other fields. "The field is thus a dimension that is neither subjective nor objective, a dimension that forms the basis from which subject and object emerge" (Francesetti, 2020, 47). Since contact is the first reality, individuals are never detached from other people, current situations, or their 'habitat'. At the same time, fields do not have a life of their own, lurking to ambush unwitting passers-by. While measurable field elements such as geographical realities, environmental conditions, (physical) affordances, social opportunities, and financial limitations do exist, fields are nothing without the persons anchored in them. "Fields cannot be spoken of properly as existing in themselves, in nature, apart from a co-constitutive human subjectivity, and it is this philosophical tenet that justifies gestalt therapy's reverence for first-person human experience" (McConville, 2001, 201). In my view, fields encompass both phenomenological experiences and real (physical) circumstances. A person's subjective impressions and sensations are not arbitrary, nor constructs rising from some kind of interior processes, nor mere *re*actions to exterior forces. Consequently, I find the term organism no longer useful. It is an all too biological concept, as Wagner (2019, 107) rightly suggests. The idea of an organism surrounded by a field is based on the outdated Cartesian-individualist paradigm. It repeats the old dualistic tradition. In this respect, it cannot provide orientation for therapy in the liquid modern age.

3.2 People are of the field, not in it

Perls, Hefferline and especially Goodman rejected ideas which attributed life to individuals independent of their environment. But it was only later publications that specified a gestalt therapeutic field theory. "People are not born with a separate essence that later interacts with an environment, but the individual and environment are a whole out of which the external and the personal aspects are differentiated" (Yontef, 1993, 360). He rightly insists on a crucial linguistic difference: "Being *of a field* is not just being in a field. '*In* the field' defines the organism or object in absolute terms, i.e. outside the field, and then adds the field for context" (ibid., 300). While the first phrase indicates a thorough field perspective, the latter view is still based on the old individualistic paradigm. Yontef continues,

"People are of that field and are of the organizing and determining force of the field. The psychological field does not exist apart from the people; people do not exist apart from the field. It is not a case of simple relationship between a separate individual and an external environment. The individual is only defined at a time by the field of which he or she is a part, and the field can only be defined via someone's experience or viewpoint. The distinction between of-a-field and in-a-field is often missed." (ibid.)

The field and its structural elements cannot be separated from each other; the poles and forces are not only *in* a field. Poles and forces are not different entities encountering each other *in* a field. Together they constitute a structured field. Yontef and others take up thoughts that were sketched out by Perls, Hefferline and Goodman and bring them to bear more consistently.

If a therapist can never understand a client without references to their field what, then, is the relationship between poles of a field, the persons? A basic characteristic of fields is their structure where its "parts are in immediate relationship and responsive to each other and no part is uninfluenced by what goes on elsewhere in the field" (ibid., 125). The field is a whole and it replaces the notion of discrete, isolated particles. The person in his or her life space constitutes a field. The 'I' is neither a mental nor a physical particle; the 'I' is *of the field* not merely *in the field*. The distinction of the preposition marks a radically different proposition. The field is a holistic, unified phenomenon, not a collection of particles that may or may not relate to each other. To clarify this difference linguistically, I find it useful to no longer speak of 'parts' but of the 'poles' of a field, just like the "positive and negative poles of an electrical field [which] are not value-laden dichotomies but belong to a unifying whole" (ibid., 302). Analogous to physical field theory and quantum field theory, Yontef describes poles and fields uniformly. Thus, the metaphor derived from physics is turned into a description of observable and experienced processes. However, an appropriate linguistic presentation of the physio-psychological field perspective remains difficult.

As I demonstrated before psychologists and other theoreticians often define the ideas associated with the term field inadequately and inconsistently. Fuchs (2000b, 12), for example, is close to a gestalt-theoretical perspective when he writes that the felt body is not opposed to the surrounding space and it is not something material, that can be limited to the space of the body. "Rather, corporeality means a living event, namely the ongoing process of mediation between the poles of body and world, which cannot be separated from each other." Although Fuchs defines the process corporeally, he makes a misleading distinction between particles and their surrounding space, affirming a fundamentally individualistic perspective. Similarly, in 1977 Petzold thought it was essential to see "the indissoluble interconnectedness with which everything interlocks" (291). As holistic as that sounds, in fact, his further descriptions of what he called the environment prove that he envisioned a collection of particles *in* the field and not a situational wholeness. Regarding therapeutic practice, he said, "Therefore, *the therapy of pathological conditions always requires a therapy of the pathological environment*" (Petzold, 1977, 297). As if these were two different options. Much more precisely, Kepner (2008, 31) points out: "But to speak of a person as composed of connected parts is not necessarily the same as to speak of the person as a whole." Neither persons nor fields are collections of singular components, parts, or particles, but a unified and structured whole. They are related to other poles by vectors and valences.

The German sociologist Rosa starts in a similar vein: "As a duopoly, I will nevertheless hold on to the concepts of *subject* and *world* because both are inescapable in a phenomenological perspective" (Rosa, 2019a, 65). The world can then be "conceptualised as everything we encounter" (ibid.). At first, this sounds like another juxtaposition, especially when he writes, "The world is that which is always already given to every consciousness as prior" (ibid., 65f). His concept remains ambivalent yet provides a vital hint. The world is real, and it appears for someone who in turn is an integral pole of that field.

Physical reality has already existed before we appear, *and* we have a specific experience of it. Yet, the so-called 'objective' conditions do not determine our subjective awareness. At the same time, our perceptions are not mere constructs. On the basis of a field-centred perspective, both subject and world are no longer duopolies, but poles of a unified field defined by contact. Indeed, people experience themselves as separate – but also as connected. In this respect, it makes more sense to see physics and phenomenology as two complementary approaches to a holistic, structured field, its poles, and forces.

3.3 A field-centred gestalt therapy is existential

When Jacobs, Wheeler and others initiated the so-called relational or dialogical turn in gestalt therapy, they did not turn away from established principles. Instead, they developed and specified previous ideas: "At the heart of this approach is the belief that the ultimate basis of our existence is relational or dialogic in nature [...] This is counter to the usual individual-istic model of a person" (Hycner/Jacobs, 1995, 6). Representatives of a relational gestalt therapy intended to overcome the individualistic para-digm. In their views, the field is defined by I, Thou and an in-between. Thus, the relational turn of gestalt therapy brought enormous progress. Referring to Perls et al., the proponents of a *relational* gestalt therapy have stated that people are existentially dependent on and related to others: "Inclusion is instead an existential turning of one's existence to the other and the attempt to experience that person's side as well as yours" (ibid., 22). But still this can mean two individuals *in the field* or two poles *of the field*. Jacobs and Hycner have rightly emphasised that people do not perceive themselves as mere individuals but always also as related to other people. The "self is but one pole" (ibid., 202) or in other words "an inherent bifurcation or polarity in the experiential field" (Wheeler, 2000, 105). I find that still too vague. Referring to trees as an analogy, the British gestalt therapist Parlett (1997, 20) writes: "As noted above, the tree and its environment cannot, and do not, exist independently of one another; that is, they have no independent existence. So why conceptualize them this way?" The realisation that human beings have never been, are not, or can ever be individual beings separate from others has long been an important element of gestalt therapy. But as long as contact is not thoroughly understood to be the very *first* reality, Gestalt concepts are still based on an individualistic paradigm.

Gestalt therapy is rooted in existentialism: "What does it mean that existence precedes essence? It means that man exists first, meets, appears in the world and defines himself afterwards" (Sartre, 1989, 11). I suppose Simone de Beauvoir would rightly claim the same for women. Many gestalt therapists emphasise that people are not controlled by destiny or some antecedent essence. "I may be influenced by biology, culture and personal background, but at each moment I am making myself up as I go along, depending on what I choose to do next" (Bakewell, 2016). People do not live out predestined patterns; they have choice. Although they are shaped by macro- and micro-social circumstances, opportunities, demands and limitations, they make their own decisions, act in their own way and form contact and relationships in their own manner. A coherent field perspective, as proposed here, does in no way diminish gestalt's existentialism. What critics of existentialism have misunderstood as (hyper-)individualistic solipsism includes an ingrained relation to other human beings, because if existence really precedes essence, "then man is responsible for what he is. Thus, the first step of existentialism is to put every man in possession of what he is, and to rest on him the total responsibility for his existence" (Sartre, 1993, 325). The same holds true for people of all genders. Human beings are responsible for *all* their actions and inaction, including the shaping of their relations with other human beings: "And when we say that man is responsible for himself, we do not mean to say that man is responsible precisely only for his individuality, but that he is responsible for all human beings" (ibid.). What the French existentialist saw as personal responsibility in and for relationships, gestalt therapists describe as life-spatial relations and intersubjective fields (cf. Hycner/Jacobs, 1995, 108).

3.4 Contact is a field phenomenon and should be the bedrock of gestalt therapy

"We speak of the organism contacting the environment, but it is the contact that is the simplest and first reality" (PHG, 1951/2013, 227). While this turn of phrase repeats an organism–world dichotomy by describing individuals *in* the field, it singles out the initial ingredient of any situation. Since people are *of* the field – right from the start and ever after – contact represents "the simplest and first reality" (Blankertz, 2012, 11). Yontef (1993, 297) states, that the founders of gestalt therapy "set forth the basic gestalt therapy notion that contact – relationship is the first reality (phenomenologically) and the organism has no meaning apart from its environment (and the phenomenological environment has meaning only as perceived by a perceiver)". Objectively observable and subjectively felt contact is the constituting first reality of any situation. From a gestalt therapy perspective, it has never made sense to speak of an individual abstracted from their real and experienced contacts. "Gestalt therapists have placed the need for contact and its restoration at the centre of the psychotherapeutic project from their historic beginnings" (Orange in Spagnuolo Lobb, 2013, 15). This focus on gestalt formation in contact and the understanding of contact as a boundary phenomenon (cf. L. Perls, 1992, 140) has been at the core of gestalt therapy from its inception. Shedding the (hyper-)individualistic paradigm clarifies the founders' approach. It is always about the whole and structured field as created by contact, its constituting poles, forces, vectors, and valences. If we stop repeating holism as a mere mantra or worse as an esoteric projection, we need to set out clearly what *exactly* we mean by the term field and what implications our ideas have for the rest of our theory (and practice).

If people are the poles *of* fields, they become aware of this as differences between them and other people taking shape, i.e. as figures emerging from the ground. The contact boundary "is the encounter between what is me and what is not me" (Zinker, 1977, 163). Again: it's a process not a locale. Moreover, gestalt therapists have never been concerned with demarcations of entities that meet like physical bodies. "The theory of gestalt therapy studies sees the self as a function of the organism-environment field in contact, not as a structure or an instance" (Spagnuolo Lobb, 2013, 81). So self is not an entity bumping into another drifting by. "What is specific to our theory is that the self is considered in a *medial position* between organism and environment" (ibid., 80f). More precisely, for field-centred gestalt therapy, self is the process of encounter and exchange between different fields creating new structures through contact and in turn altering the structure of the initial fields. Self is a function of the field. It is created through meaning-making by poles of the field. As such it is a vector of the field with specific valences. I find that a much more consistent and fruitful description.

"Primarily, contact is the awareness of, and behaviour towards, the assimilable novelty, and the rejection of the unassimilable novelty" (PHG, 1951/2013, 230). But the field is not a third dimension that is neither subjective nor objective as Francesetti (2015, 7) alleges. What we call contact boundary is not an object, an in-between or a location. It is a term used for *field processes* that constitute contact and the emergence of 'I' and 'not-I': "Contact is the recognition of 'otherness', the awareness of difference. It is the boundary experience of 'I and the other'" (L. Perls, 1992, 84). In short, the contact boundary is not *where* otherness is met, it is *how* the meeting of novelty happens and the experience of dissimilarity. Stated either in organismic or individualist-relational terms, contact is a basic human need and a physical phenomenological necessity: "Dialogue is at the heart of the human. [...] We yearn to be genuinely valued by others as *who* we are, even *that* we are. [...] *We are inextricably intertwined*" (Hycner/Jacobs, 1995, IX). Based on a consistent field-centred understanding, contact is neither a psychic yearning nor an extrinsic affordance *in* the field. It is a defining force *of* the field with describable vectors and valences. In this respect, the demand not to go out of contact, which I have heard again and again from gestalt therapists (cf. PHG, 1951/2013, 465), is quite nonsensical. People cannot not contact! "And how can the contact be blocked if there is always contact? What else, then, is blocked? My answer is that the spontaneity with which contact is made is blocked, not contact as such" (Spagnuolo Lobb, 2013, 91). Agreeing, I do not speak of contact *interruptions*, but of contact modulations. People change the way they make contact – i.e. the vectors and valences of their contact processes – based on the levels and kinds of arousal and anxiety that exist in the field (i.e. forces and valences) and which in turn are influenced by conditions, demands, limitations and opportunities of the situation.

3.5 Conclusion

Contact itself is the first and fundamental element of any field's structure. Among other things this influences the existential process of human meaning-making. As a result of real action, the figures of 'I' and 'not-I' emerge We and the world take shape for us through active engagement. Humans are self-interpreting beings. Of course this sense-making process consists not merely of intellectual or rational interpretations. It is not about opinions, values, and ways of perception alone, but also and first of all about pre-cognitive, bodily, emotional and affective processes which start prenatal, expand in childhood and continue all through life. Humans cannot help it: "We *cannot not* organise our experience [...] *our self-nature is that of a meaning-maker*" (Wheeler, 2000, 90). Part of what makes us human is the ability to create meaning, i.e. to structure our existence and form a *conscious* first-person perspective. This describes nothing other than the activity of forming figures (*Gestalten*) drawing from and shaping the conditions, demands, limitations and opportunities of the field.

Does the living human being not disappear in this "hermeneutic circle in which the field creates the subject that in turn creates the field" (Francesetti, 2015, 84)? Are real people of flesh and blood now to be replaced by pale ideas of fields? Is our real-life experience to be obfuscated by anonymous structures? I think not. A consistent field theory and practice starts from the central human experience. Contact *is* indeed the first and most significant condition, demand, limitation, and opportunity of life. "To think in terms of contact-boundary and situation and no longer of psyche, is that not a revolution?" (Robine, 2019, 194). Yes, it is. At the same time, it is the continuation of notions firmly embedded in the original concepts of Perls et al. This development of gestalt therapy theory is driven by current practical experiences. It is also preformed by circumstances, opportunities, and limitations that in the past have afforded certain outlooks. During liquid modernity, we should stop affirming individualistic alienation even if we only do so unwittingly. I have come to realise that only a method that places the unified field in the foreground of our theory and practice can be forward-looking. Rather than treating individuals and their 'inner defects' I find it advantageous to start with a characterisation of the situation as a whole. After this first approximation, the various aspects and parts of the situation undergo a more and more specific and detailed analysis. We do not treat individual patients nor should we be concerned with bipolar relationships alone. We (hopefully) ameliorate the soil of the field.

Chapter 4

The id of the situation

Atmospheres demystified

Gestalt therapy has always been a phenomenological approach: "Our experience is never of the world as it is, but of the world as filtered through our senses and our understanding of the world" (Philippson cited in Claid, 2018, 167). In practice we start from *how* our clients experience the world. For the development of awareness, that is much more pertinent than the third-person-singular perspective of scientific analysis. As first-person-singulars however, we always only perceive some sections of the field, not its entirety. "The sphere of interest is the decisive factor in the creation of the subjective reality" wrote Fritz Perls (1947/1969, 40). That does not necessarily imply that *everything* we become aware of is to hand for us, only that it stands out before the background of the total field. In gestalt therapy, we focus on what becomes gestalt for our clients and we pay attention to what emerges from the ground. Hence, we look at things in their relation to our mutual meaning-making processes, regardless of whether an impulse comes from within (through needs or interests) or from external stimuli. That is, if we look at our clients with individualistic preconceptions.

4.1 Fields are both subjective and objective

The structures of fields consist of far more than mere subjective perceptions, especially when we probe beyond conscious perceptions and mentalisations: "For our purposes we assume that there is an objective world from which the individual creates his subjective world", said Fritz Perls (1947/1969, 38). Beyond what we sense, there is always also the measurable state of the field with its specific conditions, demands, limitations and opportunities. The ground is larger, richer, and more colourful than any figure in the foreground. In this context, Perls used the example of a cornfield that acquires very different meanings from different perspectives. While a farmer may be assessing the harvesting prospects, a pilot could be looking for a place to land, a painter might revel in colours and compositions, while lovers identify an opportunity to be undisturbed. Yet, no matter if you look at the field from the point of view of a farmer, a pilot, a painter, or a couple, it always is a

DOI: 10.4324/9781003454809-5

cornfield, not a barn, an airport, a studio, or a bedroom. We cannot avoid this "inter-dependency of the objective and the subjective worlds" (ibid., 39). Every environmental field always includes measurable and observable objective aspects. Hence, awareness is achieved through *active* sparring with those realities not through passive perception, or mere reflection, cogitation and contemplation.

"The organism is part of the world, but it can also experience the world as something apart from itself – as something as real as itself" (ibid., 38). The approach to our clients' reality is phenomenological, i.e. we start from *their* subjective experience. But the connection between both aspects of a situation – real and perceived conditions, demands, limitations and opportunities – is not always clearly understood: "We may even go so far as to say that the reality which matters is the reality of interests – the internal and not the external reality" (ibid., 40). This quotation implies a demarcation of the so-called inner world and suggests a one-sided focus on subjectivity. Based on a largely individualistic perspective, Perls accordingly concluded: "We select objects according to our interests" (ibid., 41). Thus unfortunately our understanding of gestalt formation remains all too simple. From an organismic point of view the anchoring of the first-person-singular in its objective reality seems but an afterthought appearing only when a subject starts to plan the realisation of their rising needs. Such a personalistic paradigm obscures and repeats the erstwhile individualistic dualism: "The organism 'answers to' situations" (ibid., 43). While that sounds like a purely organismic conceptualisation, Perls continues: "Again we have to be careful not to presume a causality and not to say that an answer is determined by a question." What an individual perceives, feels, thinks and does is never predetermined by objective circumstances, however much they influence the processes. Yet, the centre of his gestalt approach was still the individual situated within their environment. Hence the concept is ambivalent. For an organism the conditions, affordances and so forth appear as 'external' disturbers of homeostasis while needs disturb that balance from within (ibid., 44). In this view, reality interferes with an already existing individual striving to return to some zero-point alloplastically (i.e. by adapting the environment) or autoplastically, i.e. by means of self-adaptation (ibid., 46). While this describes some field processes very well it still focusses too much on a person *in* the field.

In the interplay of organism and environmental field (if one chooses that terminology), the so-called subjective world is not an arbitrary construction at all. Reality is real: "Water wets and fire burns, whether I know it or not" (Ferraris cited in Meier, 2017, 132). For humans, the proof of the pudding always is the eating. Without references to a measurable or perceptible field, without interaction, and without real contact to reality, no self-control can succeed. This is part of our situation and that of our clients. We experience realities as resistant or supportive and their qualities emerge in contact. There is an autonomous reality that is independent of human perception and consciousness. I concur with Goldstein (1934/1995, 232) who lamented a "false emphasis on subjective experience." Using the example of anxiety, he rightly pointed out that affective states, emotions, and thoughts are often hard to understand without their field references: "The state of anxiety becomes intelligible only if we consider the objective confrontation of the organism with a definite environment" (ibid.). I conclude that some aspects of the field are objectively co-existent or pre-existent: "We have no choice but to recognise that there must be some objective, mind-independent facts" (Boghossian, 2006, 57). The demands, limitations and opportunities that arise from respective conditions of the field influence the process of gestalt formation and the actions of the individual person, which in turn changes the field structure. However, it is only when contact is considered as the first reality, that field is seen wholistically. In other words: we should not be concerned with a dichotomy of individuals and fields nor of perception and reality. The array of poles, forces, vectors, and valences comprise a structured unified field with a discernible topography. "For us, mental as well as physical phenomena are only different aspects of a unitary life process. That, what is usually described as anxiety is only the side of the process that presents itself from the psychological aspects" (Goldstein, 1934/1995, 232f).

Any field consists of real and experiential forces, not external reality and internal processing. During our entire life that is the case. "The possibilities of this environment and its obstacles are determined not by the child's needs but by the fact that it lives in a social field of forces that manifest themselves primarily through the will and demands of the parents" (Wollants, 2012, 29). Developmentally, the physical as well as relational demands, limitations and opportunities are of great importance. Primarily these include muscular and coordinative potential, gravity, and the weight of objects. In this reality of available or unwieldy objects, children learn to move and handle them and themselves. This requires physical and affective-emotional-mental skills, which they acquire by testing, training, and modulating their own physical actions. The behaviour of parents and other relevant caregivers – and a child's experience thereof – represents additional dimensions of affordances. Others' actions and reactions, their support or resistance, their demands, encouragements or restrictions either expand or limit a toddler's self-efficacy and their experience of their own abilities. "There are two general conditions that define reality as a psychological fact for the child: the will of another person and the resistance of things to the child's will" (Lewin in Wollants, 2012, 30).

4.2 The poles and forces of a field co-create gestalts

Even before birth, we humans exist in situations determined by factors beyond our control which have their own history. The world we are aware of "seems to come to us *already organised,* 'prepackaged' as it were, into the objects and events and patterns and sequences we know and see, and then take up and interact with as our given, known world" (Wheeler, 2000, 80). From these conditions, demands, limitations and opportunities, we create our existence and our essence. Thus, we create meaning. However, in developing our selves through practical action, we always 'inter'act with real things and people. Only in practical contact do we encounter otherness. Thoughts, feelings, images, associations, phantasies, or needs are not a *'deus ex anima'* that arises from some inner life or the brain. They are re-/actions that are anchored in physical and psychic conditions and in turn influence and change them. A child's immediate living conditions include for example the family structure (whether it is traditional or not, nuclear or extended), how many and what siblings live in it, and the demands on gender-specific role behaviour. This connects to the broader field: societal norms, values, and expectations. So, a child's forming of their first-person-singular perspective is always influenced by broader social conditions, such as the economic status of the family, the presence of hunger or wars, the level of industrialisation, the availability of government welfare schemes and much more. So we "can reasonably suppose that the real world in some way constrains or limits and informs our *range* of viable interpretations" (Wheeler, 2000, 87). In field-centred terms, our first-person-singular perspective is pre-formed by the vectors and valences of societal conditions, demands, limitations and opportunities as they are present in the child's immediate environment. They foster or limit how we experience the world and what we experience of it. Based on these vectors and processes, people co-create their subjective field through action, i.e. they form figures of perceptions, emotions, and opinions steered by which they then act and react. "Namely, the individual organises his or her phenomenal reality according to the primary valences – the prompting character – of the field factors" (Wengraf, 2016, 15). In contact with real opportunities and risks that 'populate' our environmental field, as children and later as adults, we develop our *personal* reality. "We have been arguing, of course, that the essence of contact is being in touch with the situation; the self-function is a function of the field)" (PHG, 1951/2013, 388). Awareness as a term only makes sense when related to an 'external' reality.

When one builds gestalt theory on the field-centred paradigm, further questions arise. What exactly is an individual in contact with? What is the otherness and how is it experienced? If we understand the environmental field only as a personal or passive imaging of reality, of objects as they subjectively present themselves, we are stuck with ideas of a self-referential, solipsistic individual (*individuum ante res*). Real contact, however, always happens when the field differentiates into 'I' and 'not-I'. *Physically,* this differentiation has been present since birth, even if a person is not yet aware of it at that stage. In fact, it is not the alleged 'inner' needs that drive the individual to move towards a pre-existent world outside. It is a unified process: "The world comes towards the experiencing subject – and the subject enters (acting and developing) the world. Some authors suggest that world relations can therefore be distinguished according to where (in the respective world experience) the primary movement emanates from" (Rosa, 2019a, 211). However, this is only the case if we ponder a temporal or spatial section of experienceable reality. When the entire field or situation comes into view, individual cognitions and actions become visible as complex, interrelated, and mutually influencing field processes. The situational demands of the field are what some call affordances. "The affordances of the environment are what it offers the animal, what it provides or furnishes, either for good or ill. The verb to afford is found in the dictionary, the noun affordance is not. I have made it up. I mean by it something that refers to both the environment and the animal in a way that no existing term does. It implies the complementarity of the animal and the environment" (Gibson, 1979, 127). That is quite compatible with the existential and experiential outlook of gestalt therapy. Similarly, the Flemish gestalt therapist Wollants (2012, 95) defined objective field conditions as the id of a situation meaning qualities, restrictions, and demands including physical circumstances. In traditional psychoanalysis, id is defined as the 'reservoir of drives' and is located in the body."

Talking about the 'id of the situation' relocates it to give primacy to the situation as the source of the experience" (Robine, 2019, 194). This idea builds on the primacy of the first reality, i.e. contact. Physical reality and individual perceptions are always the product and the raw material of co-creation: "we are both the creators of the situations we live in, and we are simultaneously created by those situations. [...] Field and situation are neither synonymous nor equivalent" (ibid.). At a given moment, in a given place and in relation to the meaning they create, different protagonists have a synthetic perception of certain elements of the mutual field. This perception "structures the context of their encounter, gives it meaning and implicitly defines the modalities of their interaction. The situation is created by the intersection and interaction of the fields of each of the actors involved" (ibid., 194f). When we stop positing individuals and environments as opposing each other, when we start from the co-created situation and when we do not split the individual perspectives from the physical realities, it becomes much clearer what the process of contact consists of. "The perception of reality is the awareness of what is, and what it depends on whatever you bring to a situation in yourself and whatever happens to be available in the situation. It depends on interest and availability" (L. Perls, 1992, 159). I find this phrasing as simple as it is apt.

With reference to Lewin's story about the different perceptions of a landscape – like that of Fritz Perls mentioned above – Wollants (2012, 76) wrote, "This difference means literally that a lion perceives other things than the things that a monkey perceives in this environment. It also means that the environment calls for different activities from the lion and the monkey."

While the first sentence provides the classic example of a phenomenological perspective, the second refers to real elements that also affect the situation. Those aspects of the situation are not constructs of a perceiver, but represent measurable conditions, demands, limitations and opportunities. Lions and monkeys are equipped with different physical abilities, their diet requires distinctly diverse actions, their survival is threatened differently, and the environment offers them dissimilar opportunities and risks. Regarding human needs, PHG (1951/2013, 404) stated, "Appetite seems either to be stimulated in the environment or to rise spontaneously from the organism. But of course, the environment would not excite, it would not be a stimulus, unless the organism were set to respond." This is co-creation in a nutshell because it describes the *dialectical* connection between the id of a situation and the phenomenal field. The field "includes the person and the environment. The two parts are an interdependent, dynamic system" (Lewin, 1951/2012, 28).

What begins during our prenatal existence, continues throughout our whole life: "every kind of social life takes place within certain limits which decide what is possible and what is not, what can happen and what cannot happen" (ibid., 206). Whereas Lewin wanted to prioritise the non-psychological factors, such as climate, laws of the land, organisations, etc., individualistic gestalt therapists often take the opposite perspective. But no matter which way we *approach* the field, "it is the stubborn indifference of the world to my intention, the world's reluctance to submit to my will, that rebounds in the perception of the world as real" (Baumann, 2000, 17). Without this sense of reality, without contact with actual objects, structures, processes, etc., all communication would lack a point of reference for the necessary meaning-making. Only through the interwoven exploration of ideas and realities do the "schematics of currently suggested ways of existence" (Grubner, 2017, 230) become understandable – for our clients and for us. The opportunities and limitations of liquid modernity are active field forces affording affective, cognitive, and behavioural patterns.

4.3 Constellations are vectors, atmospheres are valences of field

Therapy needs to address the conditions, demands, limitations and opportunities of our client's situation as thoroughly as possible. This includes physical conditions as well as the ability to perceive and think about previous experiences, values, etc. The field is more variegated, and it offers many more conditions, demands, limitations and opportunities than humans perceive at any given moment. What becomes a gestalt for us, what we sense, know, believe, and influence is but a fraction of what is present in a situation. The meaning we co-create is a mere fragment of a field's 'ids'. *What* people know about realities, *how* they perceive, evaluate and act upon conditions, demands, limitations and opportunities, is never an isolated individual process *within* an individual or *inside* their brain. Meaning is *co-created* by the poles of a situation. In that sense, mental symptoms are hybrid. Subjective mental symptoms "are constituted, in variable proportions, by both a neurobiological element and a 'semantic' element" (Marková/Berrios, 2019, 135), and by environmental circumstances. Other people are always involved because contact is the first reality: "Interactions with the environment refers to interactions with various aspects of this, including other people, noises, smells, animals, landscapes, buildings, news agents, and so on" (ibid., 134). Our clients' mode of contacting (both in therapy and in the rest of their lives) is the primary focus of our attention, not some projected inner disorders. Moreover, as therapists we cannot afford to disregard realities and their affordances because what a person perceives as reality is not an arbitrary, emotional, or mental construct. Their "inner experiences were sparked by their environment, for nothing is fully projected. Everything I see is determined in some measure by what is out there" (Zinker, 1977, 261). The insights and expressions of our clients are situational '*gestalten*' grounded in physical processes and influenced by field vectors and their valences. All conditions, demands, limitations and opportunities that are active in a situation are relevant to understanding the circumstances and can offer activators for growth.

So what about atmospheres? Are they poles of the field, too? The term has recently been popularised by neo-phenomenological gestalt therapists. According to the German inventor of the so-called 'new phenomenology', atmospheres can take hold of people from the outside (Schmitz, 2007, 13). For neo-phenomenologists, atmospheres curtail the freedom of the subject; thus they are seen as actors in the field, independent of whether anyone perceives them (for a critique see Gutjahr, 2016). But most gestalt therapists rightly question the wisdom of misunderstanding atmospheres as acting field forces: "Up to now, I did not see yet the interest of looking at 'atmosphere', as well as emotions or many other experiences, as almost things ... Why such a reification?" (Robine, 2016, 2). Of course, there is a structured (physical) field before human perception and there are constellations of objects. But gestalt formation can only happen when people are present. Subjects are the poles of a field; only they have the ability to perceive and act (cf. McConville, 2001, 200). Without a holistic view of field processes, the interplay of ground and figure turns into a chicken-and-egg problem: Is it individual monads reaching out into the world or is it atmospheres and feelings that capture them? While the latter view is hardly compatible with any form of gestalt thinking the whole problem becomes redundant if looked at from a field-centred perspective: there is no priority of either individuals or their environment. Contact is the first reality. Figure formation and the differentiation of 'I' and 'non-I' is a function of the field, 'populated' by various forces and valences.

Neo-phenomenologists claim feelings or emotions are also atmospheres, and as such they can take hold of individuals. The founders of gestalt therapy saw that differently: "An emotion is the integrative awareness of a relation between the organism and the environment. [...] As such it is a function of the field" (PHG, 1951/2013, 407). Moving beyond the individualistic paradigm, this becomes even clearer. Feelings, i.e. affects registered by an individual, do not originate within that person nor are they instigated by an outside force. "V = F (P,U) behaviour is a function of the person and his environment" (Lewin, 1951/2012, 271). The notion of feelings as external atmospheres seizing a person does not fit with either theory or practice of gestalt therapy, nor with broader research. Damasio (1999, 36) wrote, that it is sometimes apparent to us that a particular state of feeling (be it anxiousness, irritation, pleasure or relaxation) "has not begun at the moment of knowing but rather sometime before". While that first sounds like a confirmation of neo-phenomenological notions about quasi-things lurking about, Damasio goes on to distinguish explicitly between a) affective reactions ("*state of emotion*"), b) phenomenally experienced feelings ("*state of feeling*") and c) conscious emotional states or reactions ("*state of feeling made conscious*") which respond to "inducers" (ibid., 37). For him consciousness is only one element of the ongoing processes (ibid., 47). For field-centred gestalt therapy, atmospheres and feelings cannot be quasi-things *in* the field. Rather, they are integral structural components (vectors and valences) *of* the situational field.

Analysing fields, Lewin mentioned a "social atmosphere", the "social climate" and the "group atmosphere" (1951/2012, 72, 95 and 226). For him, atmospheres were "more general properties of the field" (ibid., 273). Thus, he was far removed from any metaphysical theorising. For him "psychological atmospheres are empirical realities and are scientifically describable facts" (ibid., 273f). In this field-centred view, atmospheres are not diffuse, spatially unextended and only perceptible by the felt body ('*Leib*'), as neo-phenomenologists surmise. Atmospheres are felt and measurable as real conditions, demands, limitations and opportunities of the situational field (ibid., 226). They do not mysteriously come upon us. They are another id of the situational field that can influence people and that people can influence. "All that we generally call 'mood' or 'atmosphere', into which we are brought by a certain sensory stimulus" (Goldstein, 1934/1995, 210) are physically anchored vectors and valences. As people are the sensitive poles of the field, atmospheres are sensations based on constellations. To put it bluntly: What we call atmospheres are aspects of our perceptions of a field's structural elements. That involves both physical and immaterial vectors. When we define atmo-spheres as physically real and phenomenally perceptible processes *of* the field, we view the situation in toto: "Such an understanding of affects allows for the exploration of affects (and affective atmospheres) as neither solely located in the material environment nor solely in the human body, but as emerging from the resonances between its various components" (Michels, 2015, 257). Atmospheres are field phenomena. At the beginning of figure formation, they are often only dimly perceived and at that point the way in which they 'colour' the situation remains unclear. But this is the crux of the neo-phenomenologist's quasi-matter: it references only one aspect of the situation, that is its beginning and the subjective experience of atmospheres. Schmitz and others do not trace or analyse processes of the field – they only look at snapshots. Hence, they cannot grasp the phenomenon properly. As they cut a situation into slices of experience, they reify atmospheres into actors and deform gestalt therapeutic theory (and practice) beyond recognition. Schmitz's ideas cannot nourish gestalt therapy (cf. Gutjahr, 2018).

Complicating matters even further is the fact that the term atmosphere is often used synonymously or at least indistinguishably from mood or aura. Zinker (1977, 138) for example conceived of moods as phenomena on an individual's side of the contact boundary. Once again, the fundamental dilemma of the individualistic paradigm resurfaces. The exact relations between 'outside' atmospheres and 'inside' moods remain a mystery, not because the processes are elusive but because the individualistic manner of looking at them cannot elucidate what is going on. If, however, we define atmospheres as properties of the field and vectors of the situation rooted in physical constellations, moods are what we feel of it. Both atmospheres and moods are affective reactions to socially produced constellations. Following Böhme's phenomenological and aesthetic understanding of atmospheres as bodily sensing spaces of movement, Löw (2001) develops a spatial-sociological concept of atmosphere. She conceives of moods and atmo-spheres as the perceived side of socially constituted spaces. With reference to Bourdieu, she understands atmospheres as an expression of habitual commands and prohibitions to act. Löw introduces an idea into the discussion of atmospheres that seems to be especially helpful in liquid-modern times: physical constellations are overlaid with and formed by societal ids including stereotypes and introjects. Atmospheric spaces and corresponding moods are particularly pre-structured by power. If we understand atmospheres as socially constituted constellations plus equally afforded subjective reactions to them, then it cannot be a simple matter of them being out there grabbing an unsuspecting individual. That is what neo-phenomenological gestalt therapists overlook or ignore: societal ids interfere in various ways because they are part of the holistic field processes. As contact is primary, figure formation is socially influenced right from its inception. By way of example, I would just like to point out the perceptual differences and varying attribution of meaning to natural phenomena. Cherry blossoms 'trigger' completely different reactions of meaning-making in Japanese culture than in Europe. Reactions to blooming trees are neither natural nor universal. They constitute topoi, i.e. standardised schematics of cultural imagery.

Löw aptly points to the active contribution of people to the perception and creation of atmospheres. Socially situated people co-create physical structures and constellations. Together with other people, they perceive these constellations as conditions, demands, limitations and opportunities and create their individual meaning based on jointly fabricated notions. People create meaning (including atmospheres) albeit not of their own free will, "not under self-chosen circumstances; but under immediately found, given, and handed down circumstances." (Marx, 1852). Based on this, even darkish forest atmospheres repeatedly invoked by Schmitz can be demystified. They are not metaphysical quasi-things that are loitering about. These and other atmospheres are rather attributions of meaning based on physical, social, cultural, and psychological conditions, demands, limitations and opportunities. They are vectors and valences of the field as it has developed historically as well as personally. Thus they have an effect on its structure and the processes of meaning-making. What we perceive as an atmosphere of the forest for example is a holistic process consisting of

- spatial and temporal field constellations (of temperature, sounds and noises, light and shadow, etc.),
- objects with references to each other (such as density of undergrowth, visibility conditions),
- socio-culturally encoded and traditional patterns of interpretation (topoi, stereotypes, etc.), as well as
- psycho-physical processes of perception and interpretation of a perceiver in the situation.

"An atmosphere can therefore, paradoxically, be everything and nothing" Francesetti and Griffero (2019, 1) claim unhelpfully. On closer inspection, though, moods and atmospheres turn out to be physically based and they exhibit specific structures. They can be defined and understood scientifically. They are processes of the field that can also be described phenomenologically. They are about meaning making and the people involved construct them neither out of thin air, nor are they only passive recipients: "Things perceived are not received passively in consciousness but are rather constituted by the act of perceiving" (Fuchs, 2019a, 111). Every process of perception is not something imprinting itself on our mind like a stylus on a wax tablet. It always involves activities. Perception is a holistic process, not a sequential one: "We don't *first perceive* and *then* interpret" (Wheeler, 2000, 86). The physical conditions, demands, limitations and opportunities cannot be separated from the process of meaning making. Both aspects (referred to as physics and psychology in somewhat abbreviated form) create the field.

The manner and content of active perception form constituent parts of interactive field processes. These are socially mediated, through handed-down experiences, traditions, social norms and cultural beliefs or topoi. Among other things, perceptual habits, social narratives and imagery also play an influential role. They are part of the field that is both real and perceived.

Löw's reference to power-related imperatives and prohibitions extends Wollants' thinking about the id of a situation in an important manner. While it is the fleeting nature of atmospheric impressions that initially seems to speak in favour of the term, this also constitutes the debilitating limitation of the term and its usability. Atmospheres are much more than a 'something' that people perceive. The processes of perception are multifaceted; the atmospheric content is neither a subjective projection nor a passive individual reaction, nor does it always trigger the same (or any) reactions. "The very same tones or sound waves that are able to move us to tears today may only have a weak resonance effect tomorrow, or none at all" (Rosa, 2019a, 163). How then can we grasp the complexity and volatility without getting stuck in recounting individual cases? To me, this seems to be the shortcoming of Francesetti's atmospheric terminology. He defines atmospheres all too one-sidedly, i.e. only in phenomenological (or *neo*-phenomenological) terms. His use of the terminology remains firmly within the confines of an individualistic perspective. Thus it suggests a primacy of *either* inner constructions *or* wafting quasi-thing. To come down on either side of that dichotomy answers the wrong question.

4.4 Atmospheres are being manufactured as products not least on liquid markets

Atmospheres are not just vague intuitions. Nor are they simply *given* attributes of a situation. At least in part, they are created by people – as physical and affective constellations. The therapeutic setting itself has become a social and affective trope charged with atmospheric ideas. Yet, it is based on physical constellations, such as Freud's arrangement of the couch facing a myriad of artifacts from antiquity. Published images, films, novels, etc., have also influenced the public's perception of therapy – both regarding its function and its processes. Whether we like it or not: that is what our clients bring into our practices. Moreover, the arrangement of an advantageous setting or atmosphere has been part of the discussion amongst therapists for a long time. The gestalt therapist Zinker (1977, 59) wrote, "Ideally we set a scene in such a manner that the atmosphere itself coaxes the person to do the shifting out of his internal rhythm, his inner sense of rightness." In other walks of life, too, atmospheres are being created deliberately – often to enhance market chances. In business contexts, for example, atmospheres are now seen as economically useful variables of leadership. For example, the self-styled 'atmosphere consultant' Julmi and the neo-phenomenologist Rappe (2018) claim, "Only if a leader recognises the effect of atmospheres can he or she lead in a targeted way." The phenomenon of atmosphere is well known, they claim, but a strategy on how to utilise it has so far been in short supply. Their ideas turn atmospheres into a marketable product enhancing the skills of leaders. Amongst other points, their publisher's promotional text (www.hanser-fachbuch.de/buch/Atmosphaerische+Leadership/ 9783446455771) promises the book will present techniques for specifically influencing the atmosphere and describes many examples, tips and tricks for implementation.

While Schmitz's 'new' phenomenology harks back to pre-modernity (cf. Gutjahr, 2018, 170ff), his apologists endeavour to increase the exchange value of those ideas in modern liquid markets. It seems metaphysical definitions of atmospheres are quite compatible with the hyper-individualistic pressure for self-enhancement. Similarly, some marketing experts create gripping atmospheres for advertising and sales. What they label 'resonance fields' are "widespread ideas and collective thought patterns in the audience that are accessible to everyone" (Brandmeyer et al., 2011, 5). Their technique supposedly has the "ability to locate a reference potential available in the collective consciousness and to mobilise it through an individual design for one's own point of view that has not yet been asserted in the audience" (ibid.). The authors intend to use collective ideas that exist in a society and are shared by almost everyone to manipulate buying patterns. Their ideas include archetypes, clichés, myths, and topoi. As an example for a *purposely designed atmosphere*, Brandmeyer et al. cite an advertising campaign for Tyrolean Alpine farmers' butter (*Tiroler Almbauern Fassbutter*), which used ideas, associations and the correlated feelings already present in society to promote the product. Atmospheres, I conclude, are constellations triggering common beliefs and emotions (amongst other things). They do not lurk passively and they are not phenomena happening of their own accord. They can be fabricated to increase exchange value much as other atmospheres were deliberately mass-produced in Nuremberg in the 1930s. Only Schmitz and other neo-phenomenologists, it seems choose not to understand this.

4.5 Conclusions

"Above all the field is organised (meaning it arises out of the constellation of all the energies, vectors, or influences in the field as they act together)" (Parlett, 1997, 19). This refers to the totality of field structures, including inherent power relations, distribution channels, cultural or ideological views, conditions of participation and possibilities for change, social rules, laws, and much more. Each field has its own complex structure, which includes patterned interactions, forms of communication, rules, norms, benefits, and conditions of participation. As structured constellations *of* the field, they can be analysed. Ideas about the production of atmospheres show that (1) the term is much more complex than the talk of quasi-things suggests, and (2) atmospheres can be brought to bear in different ways and in a variety of social contexts (therapy, corporate management, advertising, political mobilisation, etc.). By the same token, atmospheres are not simply given – often enough they are created. They are steeped in relations of economic, political, and social power. A thorough understanding of the term atmosphere needs to encompass divergent valences:

1 *Measurable constellations* that are created by people (e.g. in the form of the designed entrance area of a practice) or circumstances (natural lighting, trees, etc.) or interpreted in a culturally and socially preformed manner. By chance or purposefully, they create associative references that invite (re-)action.
2 *Cultural and social ideologies, introjects, stereotypes or topoi* (Miller, 2015, 5.2). This is not primarily a matter of deliberately disseminated myths or the like, but of views and patterns of perception that exist or prevail in a society.

Our understanding of moods and atmospheres does not necessarily need to be murky. But since the terms can mean everything, anything, and nothing much at all, I find them too fuzzy for any consistent use in gestalt therapy. As the aspects of creating atmospheres are often overlooked they also blind us to the influence of power in forming those atmospheres. I refrain from using either term.

Chapter 5

In contact we are being resonated

When describing processes 'between' humans, definitions of resonance are often referenced (cf. Thomä, 2016, 2). Descriptions of *physical object–object relationships* as oscillating systems are transposed to subject–subject relationships in order to describe the processes of mutual excitation. Gestalt therapists also refer to resonances (cf. Francesetti, 2020, 52–54). By way of illustration, Hycner and Jacobs (1995, 123) describe the way Martin Buber gave attention "as letting a soft tone sound and swell in himself and listening for the echo from the other side." Critics of the terminology, however, state that the use of this metaphor carries "traces of a 'mythoid excess'" (Hogrebe, 2006, 332). Others emphasise that, "resonance phenomena are difficult to explain in the context of scientific psychological theory" (Geuter, 2015, 310). Yet in phenomenology the concept of resonance "has become common to describe the kind of affectation that a person experiences in an emotionally significant situation. [...] Of course, the term is initially a metaphor" (Fuchs cited in Scheurle, 2017, 40). Of course? Is resonance really nothing more than an analogy for psychological processes without any explanatory value? What happens if we take the term as a description of observable and perceptible field processes?

5.1 Resonance is not just a metaphor

"In physics, resonance refers to the reinforcement or prolongation of sound by reflection from a surface or synchronous vibration of a neighbouring object" (Miller, 2015, 1.6). Through natural vibration, an object influences another object, which has a similar frequency and consequently also vibrates within itself. Thus, resonance is an amplified reaction of a vibratory system. It

1 is a *physical* influence of forces (waves) on the structure of another object,
2 stimulates a resonating object to activities of its own and
3 can have a feedback effect on the structure that initially vibrated.

DOI: 10.4324/9781003454809-6

Adopting a systemic view, some theoreticians have stated that resonance consists of numerous reciprocal actions by which all spatio-temporal structures can enter a relationship with each other (cf. Cramer, 1996, 14). I do not want to create a theory of everything here. What I find illuminating in the context of a field-centred gestalt therapy is that individual objects do not represent *separate* entities. They are connected to each other through real forces (waves, energy, etc.). They are *of* the field. In this respect, resonances of electric and magnetic fields describe the distribution of force effects. Resonance phenomena happen when the poles of a field or a system are in relationship with each other exhibiting echoing oscillations in their own structures or substructures. All through the field similar patterns of behaviour emerge. Resonance in this perspective is the result of a reciprocal force effect of and on the field's poles.

In resonance, people experience a harmonic consonance, an understanding beyond words, a perception of the other person without being able to state exactly how this impression could have come about. Resonance phenomena from music are often used to illustrate this, not least because they are easily comprehensible phenomena that serve to paraphrase what happens in human contact. "When two violins are located in the same room and a string is plucked on one, the string tuned to the same frequency on the other will also vibrate [...] Subjectivity is suspended to attune to the other" (Rowan/Jacobs, 2002, 80). For the most part, this is as far as such descriptions go: they *illustrate* the processes. While they can function as apt analogies, this approach misses the actual quality of field events. Moreover, when resonance is reduced to a mere metaphor, it obscures what happens and what is being experienced in a situation. Based on this, resonance is in danger of becoming a third something 'between' the human poles and somehow *in* the field.

The analogy is limited and limiting because contacts of subjects are different from those of subjects with objects. Two subjects react to each other, and their respective subjectivity is by no means suspended. In difference to the physical meaning of the word, people do not merely return the received sound but react 'with their own voice' because they are not passive objects 'to hand' as I argued in chapter 2. As contact is the first reality of the field, resonances of its human poles are clearly distinguishable from echoes. The former occur "when the vibration of one's own body excites the natural frequency of the other" (Rosa, 2019a, 282). Not only do the poles retain their first-person-singular perspective but their capacity for and their manner of resonance is an expression of their responding otherness and uniqueness. Human bodies each speak with their own voice. It is different from echo phenomena because an "echo lacks its *own* voice, it occurs, as it were, mechanistically and without variance; in the echo only what is in each case its own, not the responder, is echoed" (ibid., 286). An echo is a one-sided force *effect on an object*. In resonance, two natural frequencies oscillate, which in turn influence each other. Because of the fundamental difference between subjects and objects, the resonance behaviour 'between' people – or rather *of* the situational field – is not a passive reverberation, but an active-reciprocal, own-voice response–response process. For the German sociologist Rosa, experiences of resonance in this respect are essentially tied to the affirmation of strong valuations. "They occur when and where subjects come into contact with something in the world that represents for them an independent source of value that confronts them as par excellence important and valuable and that concerns them" (ibid., 291). In general, he distinguishes different types of resonance:

- *horizontal* resonance occurs 'between' people (the poles of a field);
- *diagonal* resonance refers to reciprocal relationships of people to things and activities, and
- *vertical* resonance describes relationships to collective singulars (nature, art, history, religion).

"Resonance means a response from others, but not just human entities, but also from objects, things, etc." (Wetzel, 2016, 11). While this may be so, in the context of this work, I explicitly limit myself to 'inter' subjective resonances. Otherwise, I fear the term dissolves into vague moods and atmospheres. Also, more research needs to be done on such a broader understanding of resonance. For example, Wimmer criticises Rosa's concept of resonance, pointing out that it does not distinguish enough between personal-direct and mass resonance phenomena. For the purpose of a field-centred gestalt therapy, I refer to *horizontal* resonance, because it accounts for the relative independence of another first-person-singular. "Resonance cannot be forced. It cannot be produced, and, for that matter, it cannot be bought" (Wimmer, 2018, 4). Due to its fundamental unavailability, human-to-human resonance is constitutive for contact with another 'I' and the emergence of self. Why is it not just another product created for liquid markets of personality enhancement? Rosa argues that commodifying another subject transforms our human desire for resonance into a desire for objects. That is self-defeating because we merely receive a passive echo instead of having a personal and active response. "Real resonance is unavailable." Rosa (2019b, 32) When we try to force resonance – for example when we encounter each other as mere actors on the market – we transform a subject into something that it explicitly is not: an available object 'to hand'. The pervasiveness of exchange value relations today and the demand for 'authentic empathy' seems to contradict that assertion. But that is an important misunderstanding: manufactured or engineered authenticity is but an echo. As such it never fully quenches the thirst. Being a sellable product, it is not meant to satisfy completely. It is designed to assuage and stimulate further demand. As such it is another element of alienation. Subject–subject resonance, on the other hand, "changes the participants through touching appropriation or encounter" (ibid., 286, footnote 271). What touches us is precisely another self's resonance, the other person's own voice and manner of response to our advances. Every person has their own melody, Appel-Opper (2018, 1) believes, and whether a common "vibration between people" (Baer, 2012, 234) comes about depends on the ability to vibrate *and* the capacity for self-response. In other words, it is all about the use value of contact.

"Resonance is first to be understood as a basic human need and ability" (Rosa, 2019a, 293), i.e. an intentionality. For a gestalt therapist that is not surprising. For example Boeckh (2019, 20) states: "the relationship as such, that is, vital affirming contact and recognition by others, is itself a central need". When we see contact as the first reality of the field, elicited resonances are essential vectors of the field. They do not end with early childhood (Oberhoff, 2009, 170). They are lifelong *constitutive* features of the field structure; they are an id of any situation. However, "A response relationship can only be established with a counterpart who is not completely transformed or appropriated, who remains alien and unassigned to us as a whole" (Rosa, 2019a, 317). Based on a field perspective, existential otherness does not create an obstacle for understanding. Rather, it is the precondition for field resonances. This "irrevocable moment of unavailability" (ibid., 295) of subjects whose vibrations constitute a subject-based response is fundamental to the idea of horizontal resonance. Individuals have alternatives, that is they can respond, resist, repel or remain silent. Horizontal resonance is about the "core of affective attunement" (Baer, 2012, 234). Understood in this way, resonance consists of mutually stimulated oscillation processes. According to music therapist Gindl, resonance is a relational phenomenon. It "means the resonance of feelings or the reverberation that feelings, thoughts, expressions of other people trigger in me" (Gindl, 2002, 30).

5.2 Horizontal resonance is an essential field phenomenon

"Human infants are particularly immature and need the longest parental care. We humans, like all mammals, have been endowed by evolution with the limbic structures in the brain that make us particularly sensitive to the needs of our children. [... This] is the foundation of our ability to bond with others, to 'relate' to others: family, horde, tribe, and so on" (Servan-Schreiber, 2006, 199 f). The ontogenetic starting point and practical necessity of human resonance is embedded in the intimate contact between mother (or other relational figures) and baby. Rosa (2019a, 85) writes, "that an embryo forms a resonance system with its mother" even before birth. Infants are never beings 'unto themselves'. Rather, from the very beginning they are poles within webs of relationships. Contact, i.e. the processes of reciprocal resonance are the first reality of the field. Some see the so-called mirror neurons as a physical basis of resonance processes (Francesetti, 2020, 51; Boeckh, 2019, 34–36). These are "neurons with a dual function"

(Baer, 2012, 336). On the one hand, they are involved in sensory-motor functions of the brain, and on the other, "they mirror processes that we observe in our environment in a kind of neuronal simulation" (Breuer, 2002, 70). By means of mirror neurons, so the explanation goes, the body language of another person is deciphered by our brain. These neurons are the physical basis for creating a mirror image of what we perceive out there within our brain. After that, specific mirror neurons become active, which make the corresponding feelings resonate. No matter whether it is sadness, joy or anger, the mirror neurons produce the same state, i.e. the same emotions within the observing person. Again, that is an individualistic perspective. Based on a field-centred approach, ideas of resonances *in the brain* are outdated. For example, the physician Scheurle (2013, 190) states, "The physical, mental and spiritual achievements of the human being, however, do not emanate from the brain, but arise directly in the interaction space, in the *gestalt circle* organism–environment. They arise *directly from the organs of movement and sense.*" As evidence he cites the circadian rhythm. Our rhythmic human reaction to the cycle of day and night is expressed through bodily processes such as fatigue – which arise *decentrally* in the body. The brain merely initiates the transitions. In this view, the brain is no longer like a control centre that sends out content-related commands for the rest of the body. Scheurle's approach takes the wholeness of the situation into account, which is in no way interrupted by an artificial inside or outside. The reaction to another person or pole of the field is not a mere brain activity, not an integrated performance of 'body' and 'intellect', but a chain of physically observable resonances perceived by an 'I'. Contact, in this view, is not 'between' entities. Rather, everything *is* contact. Scheurle comes close to seeing resonances as field processes with both physical and psychological aspects.

At any rate: both with or without mirror neurons, we cannot get around the phenomenological category of meaning making. Suppose, for example, we see someone holding a full bottle in their hand with its opening approaching the rim of a glass. This simple motor process can have a plethora of meanings. It might imply pouring, filling, toasting, spilling, sharing or, in extreme cases, poisoning. To understand the action, it is not enough to observe it or to perform it mimetically ourselves. We need context: What verbal utterances were there? What happened before? Were there observers present? (cf. Siefer, 2010). It is always about the broader field not about a more or less arbitrary section of it. Thus, the findings of neuroscience possibly elucidate another aspect of broader processes, yet they cannot replace the description of field processes. The "existence of mirror neurons is a biochemical basis of resonance" (Baer, 2012, 337). As such they might *enable* resonance. But they cannot explain the occurrence of resonance experiences in a situation nor their meaning. While neuronal firing may be the physical aspect of affective resonance processes, it is definitely part of the conditions, demands, limitations and opportunities of the field. "Mirror neurons, as I want to understand and interpret them here, form a possible neural basis and anchorage for resonance phenomena that can be observed in the social world, but they do not *generate* and *determine* them" (Rosa, 2019a, 255). The physically measurable resonance arousal is only *one* dimension of the holistic situation.

5.3 Horizontal resonance is a central intentionality of the field

"Resonance, however, becomes a *normative* concept when and where it is to be established as the standard of a successful life and thus as the criterion of a normatively oriented social philosophy" (ibid., 294). I do not think such prescriptions are helpful not least because they go against our phenomenological gestalt approach. If we were to define an ideal of resonance, this would only create a blueprint for experts to judge clients and their success in forming 'correct' resonating relationships. A subsequent analysis of resonance 'disturbances' would be, in Rosa's sense, non-responsive, 'silent communication'. It would be the opposite of resonance because it attempts to transform subjects into objects. Obviously, we should not reduce our reactions as therapists to mere echoes. Additionally, any normative definition of resonance opens the door to all kinds of esoteric Biedermeier, and to the psychotechnicians of liquid modernity. One example of this is the propagated 'laws of resonance'. They supposedly let people change their environment if they only imagine a wish *correctly* enough: "Using many exercises and successful stories from readers, Franckh shows how you can effectively and almost playfully bring yourself into energetic alignment with your heart's desires" (www.pierre-franckh.de). To claim that people can restructure the field at will, by individual decision alone, or by the power of their feelings and visualisations, is pseudo-scientific nonsense packaged as a product for self-enhancement. By the same token, the burden of failing to achieve what was visualised is being put on the individual, and the social hegemony of the liquid ideology is confirmed. During liquid modern times, fears and longings are being commercialised for marketing and for the augmentation of authenticity. They are to increase the exchange value of people. As the fictional lawyer Alan Shore says to a colleague in the TV series *Boston Legal*: "If you can fake sincerity, you'll be unbeatable!" In my opinion, this is hyperindividualism increasing social isolation and alienation.

Agreeing with Rosa (2019a, 299–316), I see resonance in the context of alienation as developed by critical theory. He defines alienation as a form of being in the world in which subjects experience their own body and feelings, the material and natural environment, and the social context of interaction as external, unconnected, and non-responsive. This is what Rosa (ibid., 306) calls *mute* responses. Alienation is the absence of resonant experiences. This definition does not resort to external sets of norms or metaphysical essences.

Humans co-create reality, their phenomenal world and themselves through practical resonances. Since contact is the first reality, they never do this detached from natural and social conditions, demands, limitations and opportunities. "The self is thoroughly socially constituted through experiences of being together with significant attachment figures – not only at the beginning of life, but throughout life" (Oberhoff, 2009, 184). In that sense resonance is a central (human) intentionality for contact "rooted in the ego and personality functions of the situation, which becomes intention when taken up by the ego function of the self" (Francesetti, 2020, 46). As such it is an essential vector of the id-function, too, whose valence points to positive reverberation, valuing interaction and response, feedback, sharing, sympathy, attention, consideration, appreciation, respect, esteem, approval, recognition, support, and understanding. By contrast, alienation is a condition that leaves this basic need unfulfilled. In the 1960s, Fritz Perls (2019, 54) wrote, "The fact is that man cuts himself off more and more from his roots. Instead of being a part of nature, he is putting himself apart from nature. He is alienating himself from his very essence." While I do not want to perpetuate individualistic terminology, I agree with the basic sentiment: "One only feels alive when one allows oneself to be touched and transformed" (Rosa, 2019b, 32). Resonating contact is central to survival and growth. It includes:

- the awareness of concrete wishes, desires, cravings, etc., i.e. their becoming gestalt,
- the selection of objects to satisfy a particular need,
- acts that serve the appropriation of objects and their enjoyment,
- the reception and enjoyment of otherness, as well as
- digesting and utilising novelty for differentiation and integration (cf. F. Perls, 2019, 25).

In this respect, resonances, defined as field forces are essential means and conditions for growth. Blankertz and Doubrawa (2005, 180) aptly summarise, "The place of nourishment is contact." People experience this and can describe it phenomenologically: "When contact occurs, it brings about an existential feeling of wholeness and joy. The ability to make nurturing contact is innate" (Salonia, 2016, 194). Less coloured by individualistic sentiments and based on a relational perspective, Hycner and Jacobs (1995, 201) state that there is "an inherent human need to meet, and to be met – to engage with the real otherness of another – and to confirm another, and to be confirmed in our otherness. This goes beyond any currently theorized self-object need." Understood as an intentionality of the field directed at other poles, resonance processes gain deeper meaning. Resonances are more than a fundamental ability, disposition, or necessity of human life. They are valences created by the first reality of contact. They are not anchored *inside* human beings who strive outwards. Humans are always in relationships. There is no possibility of *not* recognising other subjectivities. Only through others can we access and develop our own subjectivity, the first-person-singular perspective (cf. Staemmler, 2009, 70). The constitution of self depends on resonating contact with other subjects. It follows that:

1   Every 'I' implies a 'non-I' and thus also an overarching, situationally anchored 'we'. These are both physical and measurable processes as well as subjective, phenomenologically describable everyday experiences. Resonance does not take place 'between' individuals, but in a situationally constituted 'I–You–We–It' field.
2   Classical ideas of individual autonomy or authenticity are nonsensical, because from an existentialist point of view, there is no real, true or authentic inner being that needs to free itself from restrictions and introjects as conceptualised during solid modern times.
3   The therapeutic goal is not to strengthen individual autonomy or authenticity, but personal 'response-ability' that necessarily always includes social bonds. The guiding principle is a middle mode on a spectrum between autonomy and confluence.

Resonating contact is a fundamental intentionality of the field and a prerequisite for the shaping of 'needs' in the first place. Subjective relational patterns are constituted from experiences of resonance and their absence. In this view, individual impulses and social requirements or norms are not hostile to each other, like Freud's Id battling against a super-ego. Rather, the initially diffuse childlike modes of perception and behaviour are created and validated – or devalued and avoided. "Subjects are thus not facing the world, but always already find themselves in the world" (Rosa, 2019a, 62 f). There is an ontogenetic dimension to this. Only when babies and toddlers recognise the reaction of the caregiver do they learn to feel and understand what their body is signalling (Dermendzhiyska, 2020). This process does not end at any stage of life. We always need a counterpart who is physically present or who makes an appearance when we image and remember them. Dreitzel (2007, 91) calls this "*self-ascertainment through social anchoring*", which does not happen in retrospect, i.e. *after* an experience. The action itself, including all necessary perceptive processes, are components and results of resonance interwoven with other poles and forces of the field. Here, now and for next, single aspects become gestalt. At the same time, there is a wider, mostly diffuse ground of further resonance relations, conditions, affordances, limitations, and opportunities. Defining what it means to be human without these primary connections is not merely fragmentary, it misses a central quality of our existence and experience.

To feel ourselves, we need the responses of significant others, we need a resonant field. From this perspective, normative demands are quite superfluous. Resonance is not something to be wilfully created or produced.

On the contrary, when resonating gestalts cannot emerge because the field lacks validating vectors, or gestalts cannot recede into the background due to obstructive valances like shaming, anxiety is a central phenomenon. Objectification, commodification, and alienation mute responses. Those mere echoes generate or reinforce anxiety. With reference to Riemann (1961/2011) Rosa writes that anxiety and desire can be understood as the "fundamental driving forces and existential modes of being of human beings if they are interpreted as *fear of alienation*, that is, of the world becoming mute and/or hostile and of a corresponding loss of relationship, and as *resonance desire*" (Rosa, 2019a, 194 f). Following these ideas, resonance and alienation can be seen as two ends of a continuum. For me it follows that:

1   During life, resonance processes never disappear. However, "anxiety appears as an almost paradigmatic 'resonance killer'" (ibid., 206). Permanent critical appraisals of one's exchange value by self and others produce affective, emotional and bodily desensitisation reinforcing the experience of the field as hostile. The experience of pain or shame diminishes our capacity to feel which in turn reduces our capacity to feel painful vectors *of* the field – what used to be called *in others* (cf. Dreitzel, 2007, 210).

2   Such a desensitised world drives us to banish our resonances from awareness. It also stimulates the projective urge to degrade other subjects into objects of fulfilment (cf. Rosa, 2019a, 207). Reification, i.e. the tendency to treat a person as a mere object or instrument of one's own need satisfaction, describes behaviour emanating from unfulfilled valences perceived by one or more poles. Experientially "the world is treated as a mute thing, while alienation indicates the way in which the world is encountered or experienced" (ibid., 307). Objectification as such is not to be condemned, as Hycner and Jacobs (1995, 9) point out. However, under liquid-modern conditions, reifying relations based on the exchange value of human 'objects' increasingly displace resonances. People become not only strangers to each other, but hyper-individualistic conditions, demands, limitations and opportunities pressure them to commodify each other, leaving the "need for belonging" (Bernstädt/Hahn, 2010, 283) unfulfilled.

3   "Being mentally ill often results from disturbances in social resonance or responsive action" (Fuchs, 2019b, 120). Thus it is a mismatch between the person's potentials and the valences of their environment. Other people's resonant behaviours are environmental features of either an opening or restricting nature. They co-modulate behaviour. In view of the experience of refugees Parlett (1997, 26) writes, "If the 'structures of ground' (Wheeler, 1991) are dislocated, the felt continuities of the self are also dislocated." I see this as one example of a broader point. Without

(sufficient) horizontal resonance, the development or maintenance of I-, id- and personality-functions becomes impaired.

Resonances are not internal, emotional processes, but contact phenomena, i.e. field processes. In his definition, Rosa (2019a, 298) states, "Resonance is a form of world-relationship formed by af←fection and e→motion, intrinsic interest and self-efficacy expectation, in which subject and world touch each other and transform each other at the same time". With the help of inserted arrows, he denotes the direction of movement of affects and emotions respectively. While he is stuck in the dualism of individual and environment, his understanding of resonance is quite close to a field-centred outlook. When contact is seen as the first reality, resonance depicts the complex processes involving poles and forces that give rise to ever-changing vectors and valances of the field.

5.4 Field resonance and its consequences for gestalt therapy

"Neurotic behaviours are creative adjustments of a field in which there are repressions" (PHG, 1951/2013, 447). Remarkably and despite their otherwise all too often quite individualistic orientation, the founders of gestalt therapy here talk about field phenomena, not reactions of an organism! For them introjection, projection, retroflection, egotism, confluence (and possibly also deflection) arise as reactions to arousal and anxiety reactions of the poles (ibid., 448). This is a response to hostile field conditions, i.e. vectors and valances of mute communication. Apart from other reasons, the preponderance of exchange-value-based relationships act as affordances for anxiety. They interrupt and mute productive excitement. Based on a consistent field-centredness and with the help of a corresponding understanding of resonances, people's innovative and productive adaptations become more understandable. In the context of learning and growth, the field develops different resonance trajectories and resonance patterns, such as "*blocked oscillation trajectories*", which arise "as soon as certain themes, certain feelings resonate or as soon as a certain intensity of encounter is reached" (Baer, 2012, 237). This fits with individualistic gestalt therapy ideas about contact interruptions where people learn "organismic reorganisation" (F. Perls, 1947/1969, 72 f). The field adapts to limiting vectors and modulates (or mutes) the vibrating vectors.

Due to liquid conditions, demands, limitations and opportunities, *all* phases of the gestalt therapy contact model are interspersed with aspects of resonance and alienation:

• In *fore-contact,* the perception of desires, needs, intentions, etc., is influenced by introjects, culturally preformed (atmospheric) topoi and liquid-modern exchange value expectations.

- During the phase of *orientation/reshaping*, non-market-conforming behaviours are deflected, their fulfilment is necessarily retroflected, and what is then considered appropriate constitutes a projection, because possibilities remain defined by perceived market opportunities.
- In *full contact*, standard products are consumed; this involves the 'enjoyment' of commodified subjects. Egotism, the experience of not experiencing anything new is a thoroughly fitting reaction to echo products. It induces desensitisation vis-à-vis real otherness.
- During *post-contact*, satisfaction cannot become prevalent because consuming objects rather than meeting subjects cannot still the hunger for resonance. The excitement does not decrease but instead leads into another fore-contact with other products that promise gratification and thereby stimulate buyer behaviour.

Based on a consistently applied field theory and under the conditions of liquid modernity, we need to improve our gestalt therapeutic understanding of contact. Starting with the contact phases as defined by F. Perls et al. (1951/ 2013, 400ff), the gestalt contact model emphasises the emergence of 'inner' needs and their satisfaction on the outside. Instead of assuming reciprocal resonance processes, the model focusses on '*aggredere*' actions, i.e. on activities initiated by the organism. Referencing external 'disturbers', it defines a homeostatic balance. This antecedent equilibrium is then seen as the starting as well as the end point of both excitation and an individual's behaviour (cf. F. Perls, 1947/1969, 31ff). But "'normality' is not what healthy persons aspire to" (Wollants, 2012, 40). By that token, the assumed balance no longer seems to be a sufficient point of reference. An organismic or personalistic approach is no longer sufficient to understand therapeutic processes. Due to the complex effects of validating resonances and falsifying reactions *of* the field, I come to a similar conclusion as Wollants (ibid., 55): the "Cleveland developed model [...] provides us with an inaccurate and normative description of contacting processes as being initiated by a need-sensing individual and ending by withdrawal from the ongoing contact." When resonating contact is the first reality resonances permeate all phases of contact, making the whole process a much more complex operation than hitherto conceptualised. The German gestalt therapist Boeckh (2019, 137) concludes, "While the concept of ego–hunger–aggression is suitable for the ego–it aspects in the contact process, it seems to me to be of little use for the person-to-person encounter." The current contact model seems to be limited to I–It forms of contact, that is to perceptions and the subsequent utilisation of available objects by subjects acting on their 'inner' needs. As I have argued in chapter 2, subject-to-subject-encounters (I–Thou) are in an entirely different category. From that perspective, the current contact model seems to be overly personalistic and individualistic. "It reinforces the already existing tendency to see the individual as the initial source of all contact and to neglect the demand characteristics of the environment" (Wollants, 2012, 55 f). Based on a consistent field-centredness, our description of the contact process needs renovation.

My field-centred understanding of resonance integrates definitions by the British sociologist Miller (2015, 8.4):

1   Resonating contact is the first reality of human life. It is an experience created in the moment, as a temporary, ad-hoc, or fleeting form of meaningful association. It is related to broader field forces of now-for-next.
2   Resonance with otherness (i.e. another subject) is a central intentionality or vector of the field that aims at growth not equilibrium.
3   Resonance is a fundamental and important part of everyday experience; it is part of anyone's phenomenological awareness (if not necessarily of one's consciousness) right from the beginning of life. Experiences of resonance and alienation alternate, depending on the modes of contacts available.
4   Resonance is an emotional connection based on appeals to sameness or common human experiences. Without this feeling of 'sameness', or if appeals to common experiences fall flat, then one can speak of dissonance, in which common experience and understanding is replaced by fragmentation, uncertainty, anonymity and atomisation. In other words: resonating contact is a counterpoint and antidote to alienation because it introduces calming valences in the otherwise agitated ground.
5   Resonance is embodied and experienced in physical co-presence. Interactions of bodies, gestures, and mutual physical engagements affect real-life situations; resonance is not a merely emotional, mental or felt body process (see chapter 6).
6   Resonance is co-created through processes akin to notions of feedback or reverberation in the physical sciences. Resonance is a vector of the field with distinct valences.

"The resonance metaphor emphasises meaning, as an ephemeral process which occurs in here and now contexts" (ibid., 4.10). Only, that process is neither ephemeral nor a mere metaphor. As a description of contact processes, the term completes and complements gestalt ideas about contact. Based on a paradigm of ubiquitous resonances, individualism is overcome and new perspectives – as well as questions – arise.

5.5 Conclusions

Hartmut Rosa's core thesis is, "If acceleration is the problem, then resonance may be the solution" (Rosa, 2019a, 13). This has attracted considerable criticism. "Anna Daniel, for example, points out that the nuclear family and the private environment are also permeated by power and competition and are related to capitalist relations of production" (Wimmer, 2018, 4). I agree – but this is not the focus here. The lives of our clients are permeated by the affordances of liquid markets, the dominance of exchange value relations and the hegemony of hyper-individualistic ideologies (cf. Grubner, 2017, 49). Hence, people nowadays peddle their entire self. How, then, does gestalt therapy reflect this situation in its theory and practice? What goals does it formulate? Which ideals does it emulate? Resonances as well as the desensitisation to resonant impulses or vectors modulate contact. They either counter alienation or mobilise anxiety in the face of novelty. I would like to rephrase Rosa as follows. **If alienation is the problem, then resonance may be a fundamental element of the solution**. Since the pressure of liquid social environments is to authentically present exchangeable I-, id-, and personality-functions, resonances provide an antidote against the conse-quences of alienation, such as narcissism, alexithymia, depression, burn-out, phobias and anxiety.

The founders of gestalt therapy aimed to strengthen personal autonomy vis-à-vis the intrusive affordances of solid modernity. Now, under altered conditions, this subversive individualism is no longer a silver bullet. Although Henning (2015, 201) – with explicit reference to Rosa – may not have meant it that way, I agree with him: "More autonomy is no longer an effective antidote here, because resonance cannot be forced." Although resonance cannot be commodified there are quite a few substitute products being marketed. Therapy is one of them. Since people are not mere objects, the need for recognition is not a need like any other, that "I can satisfy by corresponding *aggredi*, but it presupposes the other person as a subject. If the other person becomes the object of one's own need satisfaction, their attention is no longer recognition" (Boeckh, 2019, 65). The German gestalt therapist proposes to add a social function of the self (ibid., 98) to the list of I-, id-, and personality-functions. While I agree with his sentiment, I do not think a mere plus one helps. Resonance is not something that people *should do* or need to learn. They already have a natural tendency to resonate – unless they were and are discouraged from it. In the sense of resonant contact, Boeckh's social function permeates the established functions of self.

Chapter 6

Grounding resonance

The physical and felt body

Everyone has and is a body. This affords our unique first-person-singular perspective because it appears to confirm a separateness from each other and the ideas of individualism. In the previous chapter, I defined resonating contact as the first reality of life and a ubiquitous intentionality of the field. That raises further questions: How does the vibrating resonance of a subject, this "affective knowing about the world" (Wollants, 2012, 7) come about? How do resonant vectors of the field disperse and affect the poles, i.e. people? Can we only guess, interpret, conclude, compute, and intuit another person's awareness and experience (cf. F. Perls, 2019, 46)? Is that really all we can do? The phenomenologist Zahavi (2007, 69) assumes that humans – unlike bats – have physical similarities. Thus, we share the processes of experience. On that basis we can draw analogies. Yet, he says, we can only extrapolate probabilities. Once again this is a limitation set up by the underlying paradigm of individualism (see chapter 2). If we assume an inner and outer world, it would only be our head analysing another person's body. Some gestalt therapists, seem to agree. So our *physical body* ('*Körper*') and *felt body* ('*Leib*') only deliver the necessary raw data for our brain to process and then initiate subjective resonance?

6.1 We make contact through the physical and felt body

"Sartre as well as Husserl and Merleau-Ponty have pointed out that the felt body is not just one object among others. Its mode of appearance is fundamentally different from ordinary objects" (Zahavi, 2007, 61). In this respect, one's own body is fundamental in the self-experience of every human being. What we feel of our bodies anchors us in the biological and physical conditions, demands, limitations and opportunities of our environment. Our own bodies are never objects like others and they are not experienced as such (ibid., 61). My body is part of who I am, how I present myself and how I perceive otherness. In literature on gestalt phenomenology, too, it is repeatedly pointed out that "the experience of our corporeity is not that of an object, but rather of our way of inhabiting the world" (Galimberti, 1989,

DOI: 10.4324/9781003454809-7

11 quoted in Spagnuolo Lobb, 2015, 21). Our bodies are not simply 'to hand' and yet they are physical objects. Our own body is always felt intimately. It poses real limitations and offers opportunities for existing, experimenting and experiencing: "Every emotion, then, expresses itself in the muscular system. You can't imagine anger without muscular movement. You can't imagine joy, which is more or less identical with dancing, without muscular movement" (F. Perls, 1969/1992a, 84).

Unfortunately, some authors use the terms 'body' and 'felt body' without any clear differentiation. Appel-Opper (2017) for instance uses the word body 99 times and felt body two times. Walch (2016) mentions body 47 times and felt body 28 times. In both examples the meaning of the term seems to be interchangeable. Rosa (2019a, 68, 83, 132f) seems to understand felt body as part of the subject, while he conceives of the body as a "'medium' or 'mediator' between the (reflexive) self and the world" (ibid., 144f). He points out that body and felt body are in no way separable, that neither of them can do without an inherent reference to the other. Still, this merely repeats the Cartesian notions of an individual *in* a field with inner experiences and outer means of contact. Also, Rosa's use of the two terms seems somewhat arbitrary: "A non-bodily reference to the world is not conceivable because even 'purely mental' or reflexive intentionality is ultimately conceivable only as embodied intentionality" (ibid., 146). These findings are by no means representative in the sense of an empirical study. However, they shed an interesting light on the prevalence of linguistic and semantic confusion – not exclusively among German-speaking gestalt therapists.

For some gestalt therapists, the term body describes the physical aspects, while felt body refers to the somatic experience (cf. Petzold, 1996; Staemmler, 2003). While that may sometimes be a helpful distinction it is not universal: "That which is sensually perceived could be called 'corporeal' and that which is sensed and received in the area of one's own body as belonging directly (non-sensually) to one's own being could be called 'corporeal'", opines Schmitz (1989, 5). Unfortunately that splits the holistic field and segregates felt body and body as two separate entities (see Matthies, 2015, 92). Schmitz (2011, 5) himself concedes the point when he says, how the motor-based body scheme "steers the body anchored in the felt body, I do not know." That is peculiar, especially since so-called 'new' phenomenologists find it impossible to describe their idea of incorporation ('*Einleibung*') without falling back on *physical* processes (see Matthies, 2013, 84). In contrast, I agree with gestalt therapist Kepner (2008, 15) who says, "In looking at the person from a holistic standpoint, we must recognise that much of our feeling life involves somatic experience." Based on a consistent field perspective, a separation of *physical* and *experienced* body makes no sense at all.

"A human exists only as long as the body lives organically", Husserl wrote (Alloa/Depraz, 2012, 18). Contact through physical and felt contact with otherness is primary for human life; it anchors the first-person-singular in reality. First and foremost, my body, its physical constitution, its changing demands, limitations, and opportunities are a lifelong part of my situational id. It influences how I perceive my environment and how I may (re-)act. Whatever individual beliefs, wishes, or fantasies I hold, they cannot change the course of my physical aging process and nobody is able get past one fundamental reality: death is not a postmodern narrative. The inevitable fading of the first-person-singular is a reality and part of human experience. All through life, the eventual extinction of subjectivity remains an acute possibility and part of a person's ground, troubling it sometimes more and sometimes less. Especially during pandemics and wars, one's own demise becomes gestalt, elicits fear, and often enough interrupts figure formation. As gestalt therapists we cannot abstract from physical conditions because we aim to be aware of the totality of the situational field. The physical body, *and* what people experience of it, are our unavoidable reference point.

6.2 Not least in liquid modernity, splitting body and felt body hinders our understanding of suffering

Our clients suffer from physical and felt-body effects of alienation both from other human beings and themselves. This is not at all surprising as liquid modern society is based on the constant taxation of individualistic exchange value and forms of contact that produce mute resonances. Consequently, neoliberalism does not leave the human body untouched either. By separating the two concepts and focussing on or even mythologising *felt* bodies, we stand in the way of our own understanding of both the real processes and the modes of experience. Labourers who were exploited in early capitalist modernity have now become 'human capital' – with specific physical consequences. Increasing social pressures for shaping one's physical appearance and attractiveness afford physical armouring. The pervasive terms of market relations that induce insecurity and fear, trigger creative protective adjustments such as introjects, retroflections, and projections. Due to the hegemony of hyper-individualistic ideologies, people dull down or desensitise themselves – i.e. they reduce their ability to contact and resonate – in order to increase their own exchange value. Amongst other issues, our clients do their level best to avoid *Angst* resulting from the burden of trying to be whatever the markets demand. Referring to Bourdieu (1982), Müller (2008, 46) writes, "The body not only produces, reproduces and reflects corresponding habitus forms, it is itself structured and structuring structure." Liquid modern habitus forms are to be flexible and changeable above all else. Hence the increase of cosmetic surgery, etc., is to alter the body with its predetermined conditions, demands, limitations and opportunities. Thus the body is always an expression and result of lived relationships and of social (power) relations. Social affordances are being inscribed in the body as habitus. With reference to Norbert Elias (1980), Geuter (2015, 11) speaks of "affect-motor self-compulsion apparatuses". As such they enable or hinder and limit our forms of perception and expression.

Necessarily, the body and how we see our own body is a central object of liquid-modern adjustments and ideology. Referencing only felt body stirrings obfuscates these physically real *and* phenomenally experienced circumstances, affordances, opportunities, and limitations. If we merely acknowledged what our clients feel of their bodies, we would exacerbate current alienation processes. The so-called 'entrepreneurs of their selves' are pressured to use their own "body as a resource" (Geuter, 2015, 10) not only as a source of physical or mental work performance. Our clients (as much as we ourselves!) are under pressure to treat their bodies as objects and to commodify them. In as much as human bodies are judged according to their exchange value, subjects indeed are pressured to become available objects of exploitation. Especially in relation to therapeutic processes, this should not be lost sight of, because in the experience of our clients, *socially produced* dislocations become *felt individually* (Müller, 2008, 85). Ignoring that we would only coax our clients onto preselected (neoconservative) pastures.

6.3 Science and phenomenology are best used as complementary approaches to unified fields

"Our language supports the notion that our body is an object: something that happens to me, rather than the 'me that is happening'" (Kepner, 2008, 7). In liquid modern times, that is not just a fallacy of linguistics but part of the alienation process. Yet, the body remains the primary condition of human life; marketing efforts notwithstanding, it never is a commodity like any other. It is the indispensable medium for resonance and contact. Therefore, therapists in particular need to understand and define their own terms precisely. How is the felt and physical body related as part *of* the field? "The mode of relatedness in the natural sciences is the I–It mode of subject-to-object. The mode of relatedness in the human sciences is the I–Thou mode of subject-to-subject" (Hycner/Jacobs, 1995, 217). As accurate as this description of the two approaches to a field may be, a strict separation is not helpful. Both types provide access points to the same situation either as observable, 'objective' field factors or as 'subjective' experiences of a field's first-person-singular. Humans are always situated and that always "takes place physically and psychically at the same time" (Geuter, 2015, 2). A gestalt therapy of the field needs to take this into account, integrating natural science and psychology. The idea is not a new one. Already in the 1930s Goldstein (1934/1995, 18f) wrote that any attempt to understand life from the point of view of the natural science method alone would be fruitless. "The holistic method cannot exclude any experiences of one kind or the other. Both belong to human beings and must be evaluated in their relevance for human existence".

With reference to a parable about the properties of a table by the British astrophysicist Eddington, Palzer (2016) writes, "So it's about the table of physics and the familiar of everyday life: one object, two worlds." Fritz Perls (1947/1969, 220) stated something quite similar, "Scientifically the table has a different meaning from the practical one." Both authors speak of *a physical object*, which at the same time is *an object 'to hand' for someone*. Describing a field-centred gestalt therapy, I find it useful to consider natural science and phenomenology as complementary perspectives: "maybe you can have it both ways. Both natural and phenomenological perspectives provide useful explanations and understandings. Both are necessary for the full picture" (Miller, 2019, 97). The Danish physicist Bohr saw those different perspectives "as mutually exclusive and complementary aspects of the same reality" (quoted in Frambach, 1996, 57). The principle he established, states that two methodologically different observations or descriptions of a process or phenomenon, exclude each other, but still belong together and complement each other. The modern understanding of light as a dualism of waves and corpuscles serves as a physical example of this idea. The two descriptions are contradictory and cannot be explained by the laws of classical physics. But in quantum physics, waves and particles are situated in a complementary whole. The opposites do not dissolve or cancel each other out. Rather, they are regarded as different access points to the same field. Science and phenomenology are not in competition – or at least they don't need to be. Rather they complement each other. Rooted in an individualistic perspective, Damasio (1999, 82) came to a similar conclusion: "The study of human consciousness requires both internal and external views." The psychologist Tschacher also advocates a reciprocal approach to the processes of the field: "It is necessary to look at the processes of thinking and acting from both perspectives, from the *first and the third person point of view* at the same time" (quoted in Storch et al., 2006, 33f). Science and phenomenology in this respect are complementary ways of accessing the situational reality of the field. Based on a field-centred perspective, this duality can yield optimal results. The focus of attention then is the whole field not only the individual (phenomenology) *or* the environment (natural science).

In a similar sense and with reference to Sonntag (1988, 103), the Austrian psychotherapist Grubner (2017, 168) speaks of a "constitutive 'state of suspension' between the natural sciences and the humanities". Insofar as gestalt therapists start from a unified and holistic field and not from individual particles *in* the field, the physical body and the felt body merely represent different perspectives on the same situation. A field-centred approach needs this complementarity of perspectives. To put it more poetically, the "measured heart of the ECG ('body') and the sensing heart ('felt body') are two different and distinguishable aspects of human beings" (Baer, 2012, 30). If we disregard situational unity, for instance by localising psychological problems within human beings instead of recognising them as field phenomena, we isolate individual aspects of the totality. Consequently, we only gain a lopsided view of phenomena, causes and effects. Gestalt therapists, in particular, should be concerned with the whole field. Although we speak of physical and psychological phenomena, "we must always bear in mind that, in doing so, we are dealing with data that have to be evaluated in the light of their functional significance for the whole" (Goldstein, 1934/1995, 264). All factors, poles, forces, vectors, and valences of a field are relevant for therapy. "Only through analysis of the interactional totality of the outer and inner field do the reasons become clear just why a certain pattern, a certain action appears as a 'good gestalt'" (ibid., 292; similarly: PHG, 1951/2013, 94). Seemingly opposing views are not only useful for understanding field processes but necessary in my view. The situational field can neither be defined exclusively in physical terms nor is it merely a subjective construct. Hence we need to consider all relevant conditions, "regardless of whether they are experientially present for the person concerned or not, as well as all those extra-psychological facts that obey extra-psychological laws, such as physics, sociology and economics, insofar as they influence behaviour at present" (Lohr: Introduction in Lewin, 1951/2012, 31). As the field is a functional whole, we need an approach that matches it.

6.4 Resonant contact is physically embedded and a felt intentionality of the field all through life

The human intentionality for resonance I described in the previous chapter is physically anchored. What the poles of a field experience is fundamentally based on the range of our senses (cf. Zinker, 1977, 83). However, due to manifold modern technologies (electronic microscopes and telescopes, deep-fake videos, anonymous trolls in global chats, social bots, etc.), socially produced threats are decoupled from our individual senses. Invisible viruses, war images on television, and the menace of global environmental collapse are largely inaccessible to the immediate motor-sensory experience. Hence, these developments contribute to the alienation of people from themselves, others, and their physical environment. They trigger either complacency or uncertainty and fear. At the same time, people remain physically grounded in social situations even when they sit alone in front of a computer screen. They still (re)act resonantly; physically too. While the quantity and quality of perceptions may be reduced, "embodied simulation" (Gallese in Wollants, 2012, 78), i.e. physically grounded modelling processes, still take place. To gestalt therapists this should come as no surprise. Contact is being modified due to changing valences of the field while there is no such thing as a disappearance of contact or resonance.

Ontogenetically, contact is the first reality. The physical ability to understand other subjects is a basic endowment of human bodies (cf. Kohut, 1981a, 129). Infants recognise their first primary emotions (joy, sadness, surprise, etc.)

36 hours after birth (cf. Staemmler, 2009, 101). Because babies or young children need to understand the reactions of their caregivers to survive, they have the (physical) ability to perceive what their caregivers communicate emotionally. Children are "per se *resonant beings* [...] who cannot avoid experiencing the world as responding" (Rosa, 2019a, 605). The reason for this lies not in a metaphysically based human essence, but in situational affordances and physical necessities. This fundamental nature of coordinative events between caregiver and infant was already mentioned in chapter 5. Here I would like to address the corporeal nature of those processes. As contact is the first reality, resonant reactions are *physically based, affective-phenomenal resonance processes*. Hycner and Jacobs (1995, 218) describe just that when they write, "The emotional attunement establishes both a mutual system of physiological and emotional regulation, and also embeds the infant in a web of relatedness, without which a sense of personal selfhood cannot form."

Significantly, early childhood resonance is always more than a passive identification of relevant caregivers' emotional states. By way of motor-sensual contact, humans learn something (new) about themselves and gain a perspective of themselves. To put this more pointedly, the perception of otherness is always also about ourselves. Our I-, id- and personality-functions develop because of bodily resonances (cf. Cocozza, 2018). Children's own feelings and states of arousal only become understandable to them through the *physical actions* of caregivers and the *physical and felt reactions* of their own body. Perceptions, states, affects or feelings only become part of a child's experience through the validating responses of caregivers. Conversely, the interactive activities of an infant elicit resonances by caregivers either in the form of support and validation or they are repelled, punished and shamed. In both instances, these processes constitute self-assurance (or a meaningful lack thereof) through social anchoring. As children, human beings experience that their actions and their being have value for others – or not. Either experience then becomes an embodied part of the subject's personality- and ego-functions. The experience is stored in the physical and felt body. "Indeed, it could be argued that on resonance of movement and feeling stemming from people's mutually attentive engagement, in shared contexts of practical activity, lies the very foundation of sociality" (Ingold, 1993, 160). Since contact is the first reality, individualism's precious 'I' is already the *result* of previous resonances because humans are of the field through their body: "The self is not just a concept, idea, or psychic structure, but is a muscular self, a motile self, and an expressive self – self of bones and joints, of feet, hands, spine, and jaw" (Kepner, 2008, 140). The physical conditions, demands, limitations and opportunities of our bodies have a significant impact on our behaviour. When Kepner mentions touch, eye contact or spatial behaviour (ibid., 170), it is precisely these biological qualities that have an impact on the experience of one's own body and thus on the first-person-singular perspective. The body is our inescapable anchor in the world. All through life, it influences any here, now, and for-next. Emotions are situated and embodied through bodily states. When we take a field-centred perspective using both science and a phenomenological approach to the field, physical and felt body are "inextricably linked dimensions of one and the same reality" (Petzold, 1977, 341).

Infants react physically to the behaviour of relevant persons: "An infant grasps facial expressions before it reacts adequately to other visual elements" (Goldstein, 1934/1995, 235). So far, this description focuses only on one pole of the resonance processes. To ensure survival, maturation, and growth, the unfiltered expression of feelings must also *impress* caregivers. An adult's ability to be touched by pain or carried away by joy is thus also a generic necessity that is not miraculously gained when becoming a parent. Adult resonances are simply a continuation of everyone's original ability to resonate. As contact remains the first reality, the vectors of resonance never disappear even when the realities, affordances, opportunities, and limitations of liquid modernity profoundly deform the valences.

After childhood and outside adult contact with young children, the capacity for resonance also remains an essential requirement of the field. Without felt resonance vectors of the field, creative adaptation and growth would be impossible. As social beings in dynamic environments, people with insufficient resonance behaviour are existentially endangered. In a different context, Wollants (2012, 38) describes two examples for this need of life situations: "A bodily disabled person has to construct his physical environment anew in order to confront the demands of the situation he is in. Similarly, a person who suffers from mental disorder reduces his phenomenal world, de-differentiating and standardising the exchange with it." This is not just about an individual learning new skills using new tools that are to hand. By necessity, the appropriateness of behavioural changes is tested and synchronised in the real social environment. Here again the physical and felt reactions of relevant others validate or disallow attempts. Resonance remains a basal and life-long intentionality *of* the field – both physically and experientially.

6.5 Field resonances cannot be unlearnt or forgotten – but they can be excluded from awareness

Toddlers up to the age of about one and a half years react with what is called emotional contagion to their caregivers and to others. They become sad themselves and may even start crying when they witness another person's sorrow. At that age they are probably not aware of where the emotion originates. In other words, they cannot detect the origin and direction of the vector, yet they very much feel the valences. Later they learn to distinguish 'I' from 'not-I' and their perceptions gain perspective. The ability to distinguish one's own experience from that of another person is considered by some to be a prerequisite for compassion (Bischof-Köhler, 1989). Hoffman (2000) calls the next stage of development 'egocentric empathy'. Then, he says, young children try to come to the aid of the sad counterparts and comfort them. For example, they offer their own teddy bear or fetch an adult. Somewhat later in life, things become more complicated. Hoffman assumes that with the development of role-taking skills, a further increase in compassion and supporting behaviour can be expected. He calls this empathy for the feelings of others. In contrast, Hay (1994) notes a decline in prosocial activities at that age. In her opinion, helping behaviour loses the character of a spontaneous social impulse and becomes a considered decision. Children develop tendencies to inhibit the display of compassionate or supportive behaviour, although the cognitive prerequisites for effective help improve with age. In a German study, it was found that four- to eight-year-old children were more likely to express support for a helping action if the child receiving help had not caused their own distress, if they were younger and more familiar, if they had also helped others before, and if they had suffered comparatively great harm. All the children studied were oriented towards these criteria and took them into account more and more frequently with increasing age (Volland et al., 1999/2004). While on the one hand, children can understand the situation of other people better with increasing mental faculties, on the other, they learn social norms about persons who are supposed to be deserving of compassion or help and those who are not. Resonance behaviour is formed both by active and mute resonance experiences. Societal topoi, stereotypes, ideologies, etc., as represented by views of relevant persons are being digested – or merely gulped down. Display rules get in the way of an unfiltered show of affective resonance. Yet the ability does not disappear.

Newly born infants are already part of a situational field (Wollants, 2012, 23). The 'ids' of a child's life situation have a considerable influence on the experience of resonance and the development of the I-, id-, and personality-functions. Without using the term, Laura Perls (1992, 154 quoted in Wollants, 2012, 24) described the significance of resonance for social learning: "without assurance that the new move I need to make […] will meet with sufficient reception by significant others (parents, grandparents, teachers, peers, etc.) and is sufficiently in line with social and other norms in my life-situation, I dare not risk it". If a child's resonant sensations and behaviours are not confirmed or supported, if their resonant reactions are being invalidated, rejected, or shamed, they learn to not show those reactions. Instead resonance reactions become associated with fearful excitement. As such they are then eliminated from awareness. Yet, resonant vectors (or impulses) remain part of the ground even if their becoming gestalt is being suppressed. Importantly, this learning process is not only about the so-called display rules. The learning involves or affects all I-, id-, and personality-functions based on introjects about the acceptance of one's own physical and felt affective reactions. Rosa (2019a, 122) speaks of "the ability to suppress resonance as an essential cultural technique". In field-centred gestalt therapeutic terms: the impulsive, physically grounded field vectors for resonance do not disappear; a child merely introjects 'cultural techniques' to exclude them from awareness and display. Especially in liquid modern times, the formerly spontaneous impulses come under the control of market- and exchange-value-oriented rules. Saleability comes to prejudge for whom, when, and for what compassion is earned. The circle of those who are eligible for assistance is narrowed down, excluding threatening competitors as well as anyone who is unusable for the enhancement of the I-product's exchange value. However, in the face of environmental destruction, hunger, wars, refugee crises, racist or sexual violence and worldwide epidemics, desensitisation to the suffering of others cannot be called culture.

While resonant reactions are physically and phenomenally excluded from awareness they continue to disturb the ground. The vectors and valences do not disappear. Bernstädt (2017, 11) writes, "Shame and resistance have a distinctly physical component. On the one hand, both serve to protect what is to be appreciated, and on the other hand, they often lead to painful self-limitation that needs to be loosened" in therapy. When resonance impulses are opposed by vectors of fear, the effects are felt physically (e.g. through muscular rigidity), emotionally (e.g. by high levels of anger or hate) and mentally (e.g. by strictly maintained introjects, stereotyping, racism, etc.). Still, resonant reactions remain vectors of the ground, and they continue to push towards expression. So, despite their worst efforts, people always respond to resonance offers or requests from other people. Because of internalised or introjected social rules, however, they make an effort to interrupt those resonance impulses. When such creative adjustments against unbearable excitation are executed repeatedly, they unsettle the ground and contribute to the fearful alienation from other people and oneself. In therapy it is essential to become aware (or 're-aware' ...) of both the resonance vectors present, and of the suppression of resonance.

6.6 We cannot not-express what cannot not-impress us

Analogous to the dictum of Watzlawik and others (1969, 53), I would like to emphasise: we cannot not be in contact. In his individualistic-relational perspective, Wheeler (2000, 262) formulated something similar: "We cannot not project, we cannot not interpret the meaning of a relevant field." The situational conditions, demands, limitations and opportunities may make it necessary for the individual to reject, ignore, not feel, or not display certain bodily-based resonance processes. But no one can completely banish situational affordances to resonate. Based on a field-centred perspective our understanding of others is not an individual projection. As embodied structural elements of the field, the vectors of resonance have long been real, i.e. physically measurable, and perceptible components of the field's structure, even if they do not enter awareness. We often perceive them only diffusely: "It is not necessary to intellectually grasp and learn to read the forms of emotional expression, because we directly experience the emotionality of the other in a compassionate and empathetic way" (Dreitzel, 2007, 167). Since people are always in contact, they respond resonantly. That means they acquire an embodied impression of the situation whether they follow these vectors or not. By means of such "pre-figurations" (Francesetti, 2019, 39), resonances spread through the field.

Contact is always physical and can only be realised through physical means. But contact is not created by a monadic individual reaching out to its environment. It is a sensing of resonant vectors and valences, that is, long-present functions *of* the field. Emotions are particularly important in this process: "*Feelings are bodily experienced and spontaneously mimetic and motorically expressed assessments of the organism's situation in relation to the respective situation in the organism/environmental field*" (Dreitzel, 2007, 99). Importantly, affective reactions are both physical expressions of what is felt and intentional communication (ibid., 100). The body therapist Geuter (2015, 204) writes, "Emotions not only tell something to the subject, but also to its environment. They serve to *communicate*, too." While emotions are expressive of individually perceived states, they also call on others to behave in a certain way. They generate resonance through physical oscillation processes in which the emotions and physique of the field's poles influence each other. Thus, the poles of the field co-create a common situation. Contact is always permeated by resonance experiences (including the respective physical demands, limitations, and opportunities), by embodied resonance memories of earlier situations, as well as by resonance expectations or aspirations. Regarding all these aspects, the physical *and* felt body is pivotal: "The body is the organ of contact par excellence, which collects the memory of previous contacts and enables the creation of current contacts" (Spagnuolo Lobb, 2015, 22). As we are physically grounded in situations, our bodies are the sensors for prevalent forces, vectors, and valences of the field.

Starting from the idea of a field structured by ever-present (albeit changing) vectors of contact "expression always includes impression" (Baer, 2012, 97) and vice versa. Neither the perception nor the display of resonance is possible without a body (Kepner, 2008, 144). Sensual perceptions and muscular actions, for example, are intrinsic elements of any social contact. As such there are no functional distinctions between expression and impression. Crucially, the field does not break down into processes of intake and output; both are one and the same. Even unaware body reactions relate to others and involve communicative aspects or intentionalities: "The lack of gross body movement does not imply lack of body involvement; every experiment has a strong behavioural component in it" (Zinker, 1977, 124). Going back to the physical and perceptive grounding of contact allows us to demystify the hyper-individualistic body-to-body dualism and its supposed locale of exchange, the mysterious 'in-between'. A composite focus on the physical *and* felt body allows for different gateways to the forces and poles *of* a field. Based on a field-centred paradigm, the elusive question from chapter 2 needs to be rephrased and thus finds an answer. Instead of 'How can I feel what you feel?', the question is 'How do field resonances spread?' Yet even this question could be misconstrued as it might imply that they emanate from an individualistically defined entity. But affects, feelings and ways of experiencing are not initially personal, and their communication is not an afterthought. The forms of impression are ways of communication, too. Physically perceptible, they convey something to all who are present. When these processes are no longer seen through the lens of individualism, there is no need for the presumption of mental or physical steps of dissemination. The philosophical phenomenologist Merleau-Ponty pointed out that we never understand the gestures of another by interpreting them intellectually. "I do not sense rage as a psychic fact hiding behind a gesture. I read rage in the gesture. *The gesture does not set me thinking about the rage; the gesture is the rage*" (quoted in Wollants, 2012, 110 – italics by LG). The gesture is not a *trigger of rage* – neither in the first nor in the second person singular (I and Thou). The body resonance *is* the feeling, both expressed and impressed simultaneously. Whatever we feel and sense is always physical. Body *resonance* is *body* resonance. Merleau-Ponty (2002, 72) puts it in a nutshell: "Anger, shame, hatred, love are not psychic facts hidden in the deepest depths of the other's consciousness, they are externally visible manners and styles of behaviour. They are on the face or in these gestures and not hidden behind them." Tears, for example, are the sadness, the anger, the despair, the joy, etc. Physical expressions and impressions are the process itself.

"The features are given to man as the means by which he shall express his emotions", Hatfield et al., wrote (1994, 13), quoting Arthur Conan Doyle (*The Adventure of the Cardboard Box*, 1917). Since impressions and expressions of emotions form vectors of field processes, those feelings are immediately present. Fields are structured and holistic. This begins with the act of perception: "A person perceives with his whole body, not with separate senses. To perceive is not a question of deliberately taking up a position or engaging in a particular act, but a holistic and integrated pre-reflective experience" (Wollants, 2012, 75). Persons are poles *of* the field; their senses play an *active* role. In this regard, the term perception itself is misleading, for it is neither about being impressed passively like a waxen tablet, nor is it about data flowing from one inner world via the outer world and further via the organs of perception into the brain of another 'I'. With reference to Köhler, Wollants wrote, "Sensory organisation [...] is not carried out by the self or mental processes within the self but is inherent in the act of perception itself" (ibid.). Perception itself, the emergence of shapes from the ground, is already a co-created structuring process that in turn creates communicative valences and prevents or hinders alternative figures without ever eliminating them as possibilities.

At its core, resonant behaviour consists of reacting to and acting on situational vectors through one's own body. Im- and expressions are biochemical and physically based; at the same time, it is what humans feel about a field's vectors and valences. Reciprocal processes of expression and impression take place via sensory perceptions and corresponding mimetic reactions. "The mere sight of an intense emotional expression may already cause a similar emotional disposition to resound in the observer" (Dreitzel, 2007, 169). Using different terminology, Wegscheider (2015, 7) describes a similar idea: "Encompassment is related to empathy. Someone feels, senses and thinks what another person experiences, and at the same time they are aware of their experience." Staemmler (2009, 37) suggests that people can "produce mental states in themselves that resemble the states of those they empathise with." Unfortunately, his simulation theory reiterates the individualist-relational paradigm. Consequently, he does not get beyond stating a dualistic process (ibid., 39). Geuter (2015, 310) takes a similar view. In my field-centred perspective, I would like to emphasise the processes of *co-affective* (*re*)actions to valences of the field by means of bodily contagion – both physical and felt. In therapy they are the starting point for joint phenomenological exploration.

6.7 Emotional contagion is a field force structuring situational processes

At the beginning of the last century, Scheler (1913 and 1923, 25ff) mentioned and analysed the term emotional contagion. It has been more widely used since Hatfield et al. published a book with that title in 1994. They define the process as the imitation of another person's feelings, especially those expressed through mimicry. Such imitation is a natural human tendency, says Staemmler and he describes a number of effects (2009, 103–109). This type of 'transmission' occurs spontaneously. At first it includes a "rudimentary or *primitive emotional contagion* – that which is relatively automatic, unintentional, uncontrollable, and largely inaccessible to conversant awareness" (Hatfield et al., 1994, 5). In contact, there is a constant, reciprocal process below the threshold of consciousness. Based on a field-centred paradigm, emotions can be described as vectors and valences of the field that express and elicit resonances even when they remain below the threshold of awareness. Being part of the ground they still impact the entire situation. Mimicry or imitation is the unity of sensory impression, affective bodily response, proprioceptive or emotional sensation and physical expression. Feelings are 'transmitted' mostly without volitional intention. Miller (2015, 6.6) describes this as a 'conversation of gestures', "where unconscious communication is made through gesture, stance, pause, and by which all others unconsciously and continually readjust their position in a process akin to feedback or reverberation, to create a social situation". Today, the notions of *gestural* communication between individuals need to be expanded considerably.

The flow of resonant impressions and expressions is more complex and by no means limited to imitating gestures or faces. "There is considerable evidence that people mimic and synchronize their vocal utterances", too (Scheflen in Hatfield et al., 1994, 26). Humans seem to have a tendency towards synchronicity – linguistically and vocally, too. This is not surprising, for "an infant hears his mother speak in a certain pattern; he begins to move with her breathing rhythms, rhythmic heartbeats, movements, and so forth" (ibid., 27). The immediate, complex, physical situatedness within the situational field is already present in utero. There "predominant rhythms are already laid into the neurological system" (Condon in Hatfield et al., 1994, 27) and resonant processes are swift: "people can mimic and synchronize their speech productions with others within one-twentieth of a second. For people to match their behaviours within 50 milliseconds [...] requires some mechanism unknown to man" (ibid., 28). This is not quite correct. The mechanisms are perhaps not known as an explicit conscious content or technique and they mostly happen unaware, but the practice is known to everyone.

Imitative resonance phenomena do not only take place using muscles. With the help of electromyography (EMG) – an electrophysiological method of neurological diagnostics in which electrical muscle activity is measured – it becomes clear that this is a genetically determined ability. In surveys, happy and angry faces evoked very different response patterns. "Subjects also showed an orienting response to both happy and angry faces: Their heart rates decelerated, and their skin conductance levels decreased" (Dimberg in Hatfield et al., 1994, 17). Primates are thus prewired to respond to emotional faces with a strong response of their autonomic nervous system (ANS). All physical-affective contagion processes are resonance behaviours; they form a unity of resonance experiences and intentional resonance expressions. Even subtle bodily-affective processes trigger so-called ripple effects, which spread through the field and lead to comparable bodily-affective experiences for other people. In this manner they influence the structure of the field. Staemmler mentions "multiple reciprocal empathic micro-processes" (2009, 74). I would like to put it this way. Bodily processes trigger automatic emotional resonances. They are:

- **multiple**, as they spread through different paths, forms of expression or channels;
- **field-present,** because they interact and influence the field structure as a whole, so they are neither located in persons nor in an 'in-between';
- **resonant**, because they exhibit systemic effects;

- **body-mimetic**, because they are reflections of reciprocal physical processes that influence the behaviour of two or more first-person-singulars;
- **micro-processual**, insofar as they are not based exclusively on aware reactions, but also and especially include subtle physical and felt body processes mostly below the threshold of awareness.

Hatfield et al. (1994, 48) see the emergence of emotional contagion in two steps: "Step 1: We imitate other people – when the other person smiles, we involuntarily smile back. Step 2: Our mood changes when we imitate others – when we smile, our mood is also more positive; when we 'scowl', we feel worse." This process is necessarily simplified. Resonances are different from echoes because they are not passive occurrences but active responses of a subject. They include reaction and action, impression and expression. When we physically imitate emotional states and expressions, we experience in our own bodies what others experience, without having to resort to mental extrapolations or additional empathic processes. Based on physical and experiential imitations, we co-create holistic gestalts. This is what Hatfield et al. (1994, 4) call emotional 'packages' which "comprise many components, including conscious awareness, facial, vocal, and postural expression, neuro-physiological and automatic nervous system activity and instrumental behaviours." They are holistic processes because sensation and performance are inseparable. They are functional wholes that produce aware, semi-, and non-aware relational effects. As mimetic synchronisations they are however accessible to awareness (cf. Breithaupt, 2009, 8f).

Emotional contagion processes are not at all a matter of motor-physical mirroring in the sense of simple repetitive echoes. As one critic noted, "*Experiencing is not yet understanding*" (Metzger in Wollants, 2012, 78). Indeed, resonance is not merely an imitative re-experiencing of somebody else's affects. It is the physically anchored reaction and communicative response to situational valences. Hence, resonance is much more than mere mental or emotional awareness. Rather, we feel *of ourselves* what another person feels: "This perception [of another person's feelings – LG], however, is not a merely cognitive one, but the perception of authentic expressions of feeling also triggers a corresponding *state of feeling in* the perceiver" (Dreitzel, 2007, 104). So, emotions do not pass from one individual into another nor do they grab a person from the outside. Their (physical) display constitutes vectors *of* the field and first-person-singulars present in the situation necessarily react to them.

6.8 Conclusions

As contact is the first reality, the emotional engagement with otherness is a defining aspect of field processes. Building on that understanding, there is no need to dissect the field into separate particles. Phenomenology and physics are complementary views because emotional experience and somatic expression are tightly linked. Resonance with another person does not take place in an undefined in-between, but *on this side of a person's physical contact boundary and within what they phenomenologically perceive as belonging to them*. So, resonance does not only happen *at the contact boundary*, which has been so crucial for gestalt therapists since the beginning, but *within the entire field*. Crucially that includes everything that is understood as 'I'. Temporarily, this makes any demarcation from what is 'not-I' difficult. The experienced contact boundaries become transiently blurred and the events bear traits of confluence. Through the experience and processing of resonance phenomena, the field and the first-person-singular poles present change. Regarding vegetative selection processes, Schnee (2018, 34) writes, "The contact boundary in this case is in the cell and we don't get anything out of it." Analogously, I would say, the contact boundaries are diffuse, and we *initially* get only a vague impression of them.

Our (physical) resonances are not echoes. Rather, they are impressions and reactions with one's own frequency. Physical and phenomenal resonance is the impression of another person through multiple, field-present, resonant, body-mimetic, micro-processual imitations of one's own body. Emotional contagion is not a mere transfer of information about the state of another person *in* the field, but "a very literal means by which we feel the sensations that the other feels" (Ekman in Hatfield et al., 1994, 53). Physically grounded, feelings reside neither in one person nor in some in-between. They are forces, vectors, or valences *of* the field. The Czech gestalt therapist Roubal (2019, 74) sees a 'contagiousness of depression', another way of depicting the pulling-down power of depression. "From the perspective of the situation, the contagion does not appear as a transmission from the depressed person to another person, rather the depressed situation itself is contagious for all the participants." I agree with his assessment, because I define resonances as *real processes of the field*, not merely as metaphors. Roubal explicitly refers to Hatfield and mentions a "direct pairing or matching of the bodies of self and other" (ibid., 90). Mirror neurons, he says, create a "neural image of the mental state of the other person" (ibid.). In this view, atmospheres are not entities that can grasp a person from the outside, but physical-phenomenal resonances *of* the field. Robine (1996) called that "*connaissance immédiate et implicite du champ*" – an *immediate* and implicit knowledge of the field.

Contagion and resonance processes are initially non-conscious and cannot be specifically controlled. People are probably not able consciously to mimic others very effectively: "The process is simply too complex and too fast. For example, it took even the lightning-fast Muhammad Ali a minimum of 190 milliseconds to spot a light and 40 milliseconds more to throw a punch in response" (Hatfield et al., 1994, 38). Imitation is an innate reflex. Every movement by a relevant pole of the field triggers involuntary resonances – not echoes! This distinction necessitates differentiation (cf. Oberhoff, 2009, 115):

- *Concordant emotional* **resonances** are, for example, shared laughter of young children and their caregivers. Communal feelings at musical or sporting events are also included here. The affect experienced and expressed physically by one person infects another person in that the latter copies the physical expression of the first and thus in turn reinforces it.
- In *complementary imitation*, the identification is also non-conscious and immediate, but it is distinct from the impulse of the other person or even contrary to it.

When I watch a boxer throw a punch, I can resonate by clenching my fist or backing away from the punch. Feeling contagion is always perspectival and based on non-conscious judgements, identifications, previous experiences, sense-making processes, introjects, social rules and more. The so-called interpretations of another's contagious behaviour do not happen after an activity. They are part of the initial (*re*)action precisely because resonances are not echoes. They contain *preconscious* statements, i.e. subjective vibrations of the first-person-singular responding with their own I-, id-, and personality-functions. "Perceiving is not a mere construction of the brain, but an active performance of the organism as a whole" (Scheurle, 2013, 7).

Emotional contagion, understood as multiple, field-present, resonant, body-mimetic, micro-processual imitations and physical-phenomenal aspects of resonance, aptly describes *how* resonances of the field come about: "people may come to *know* what others feel because they feel what others feel – in 'miniaturised form'" (Levenson/Ruef in Hatfield et al., 1994, 32). The (hyper-)individualistic paradigm about I, Thou and the in-between unnecessarily limits our view of field processes. Contact, this first reality, is a process initially at the boundary where 'I' meets 'not-I'. By the same token, contact involves, mobilises, and changes what we define as 'I': the personality- and ego-functions, as well as the biochemical, physical, and nervous-muscular body states. In that sense contact is a boundary phenomenon not happening *at* the boundary but throughout the self. We, including our bodies, are always here, now and directed towards next intentions. We are in contact and thus simultaneously perceive and create situational meaning together with others. Our bodies are never separate from the field, never detached from situations. From the cradle to the grave, human beings are *of* the field – of course that includes therapy.

Chapter 7

Personalistic gestalt therapy and its subsequent relational turn

"Two people sit in a room and talk, every week, for a set amount of time, and at some point, one of them walks out of the door a different person, no longer beleaguered by pain, crippled by fear or crushed by despair. Why? How?" (Dermendzhiyska, 2020). How does this kind of change happen? What factors make it possible? And even more importantly, is the premise of this quote true? Does only one of the two emerge changed? Are we therapists working *on* our clients, i.e. on the psyche of separate individuals? Even though gestalt therapy pursued a socio-critical intention from the start, its classical self-theory represents an egocentric individualism, which is a core element of liquid modern times. "In this respect, it was not only critical of a bourgeois authoritarian coercive morality, but in a certain way also stands for a core element of the prevailing conditions" (Boeckh, 2019, 134). In this view the changes of the psychotherapeutic field induced by the ideas of Fritz and Laura Perls, Paul Goodman and many more could be seen as creative adjustments to the conditions and demands of liquid modernity. Thus, we seem to "have become, in this sense, not part of the solution, but part of the system that creates these problems" (ibid., 150). If the paradigm that places the individual at the centre of the therapeutic cosmos is no longer helpful for our clients, then what is the alternative?

7.1 Personalistic gestalt therapy aims to increase awareness – of the client

The starting point of every gestalt therapy session is what clients bring with them, what moves and concerns them: "Gestalt therapy necessarily is phenomenological because it starts with the 'description of immediate experience, as naïve and comprehensive as possible'" (Koffka quoted in Yontef, 2004, 2). Since the beginning, gestalt therapy has been about the exploration of our clients' experiences, *their* (mindful) experiencing, and *their* first-person-singular perspective. From this, awareness and change emerge paradoxically: healing happens when a person no longer tries to become something they are not (Beisser, 1970). *Gestalt* phenomenology describes an

DOI: 10.4324/9781003454809-8

attitude that does not rely on the interpretations of trained therapists to analyse the behaviour of clients. Knowledge alone does not lead to change, as Zinker already lamented in 1977 (122): "We have learned over the years that a person may 'understand' himself in great depth yet continue behaving in the same dysfunctional ways." Gestalt therapists do not provide their clients with insights from the third-person-singular perspective, i.e. with diagnoses, which they then either accept and thus achieve healing, or which they reject as long as they are trapped in 'resistance'. Instead, Lewin (1951/2012, 263) described a field-theoretical view of change in relation to groups which is also relevant for gestalt therapy:

1 loosening of the previous field level, i.e. field integration, density, and complexity,
2 the transfer, and
3 the solidification of the field at a new level.

Therapists need to get into the mental underwear of their clients, as Frank Farrelly (1974), the founder of provocative therapy suggested. For me, the most concise formulation of gestalt therapy's approach is by Laura Perls (1992, 99): "I work with the obvious, with what is immediately accessible to the patient's or my own awareness." Crucially, therapy is not a fact-finding mission. It is about the phenomenological exploration of the situational field, because "description prevails over explanation, experience and experiment over interpretation" (ibid., 95). The goal of gestalt therapy is awareness, i.e. a thorough exploration of the field. Therapy is not a mere mental process because its very success depends on the client experiencing something relevant (cf. F. Perls, 2019, 39). Awareness includes and entails meaningful action.

The founders of gestalt therapy started their theory and practice from individual needs that become gestalt as natural unhindered expressions of life: "Identification with organismic needs is originally effort-free, but, alienation is not" (F. Perls, 1947/1969, 150). Any 'normal' fulfilment of needs is achieved without a *surplus* expenditure of energy, they believed. Of course, an affective-emotional arousal in the form of aggression is necessary both for orientation and full contact with those objects that fulfil the needs. In this perspective, gestalt therapists focus on the disruption of arousal and the obstruction of satisfaction: introjection, deflection, projection, retroflection, egotism, and confluence. In a personalistic perspective, such avoidances are reactions to previous anxiety-inducing conditions. They are repeated in the here and now as behaviour designed to eschew individual pain. The driver is the "fear of allowing the arousal to flow into spontaneous action" (Bernstädt/ Hahn, 2010, 149). Originally, however, these 'disturbances' had a useful function for the individual. Gestalt therapy calls them creative adaptations. They are an individual's strategies for dealing with emerging conflicts between 'inner' needs and intentions on the one hand and 'outer' conditions, demands, limitations and opportunities of the environment on the other. "In order to avoid conflicts – to remain within the bounds of society or other units – the individual alienates those parts of his personality which would lead to conflicts with the environment. The avoidance of external conflicts, however, results in the creation of internal ones" (F. Perls, 1947/1969, 148). The after-effects of these creative interruptions of contact are ambivalent. On the one hand they allow individuals to cope with fearful situations. On the other hand, they "throttle spontaneity as well as self-responsible powerful action" (Bernstädt/Hahn, 2010, 149).

7.2 Gestalt therapy has always had a focus on bodies – those of our clients

"The body is the locus of gestalt therapy" (Kennedy, 2003, 78). In the work of Laura and Fritz Perls, the *practical* inclusion of bodywork played an essential role. They repeatedly directed their clients' awareness to their breathing, non-verbal communications, muscular tensions and "somato-neurotic resistances" (F. Perls, 1947/1969, 155). Furthermore, gestalt therapists and their clients often experiment with expressive movements in order to experience (new) possibilities of being in the world. Unlike other body-oriented forms of therapy, however, gestalt therapy is critical of ideas about prescribed changes. Instead, clients are asked to increase their awareness of what is happening at this very moment (cf. Kepner, 2008, 53). A few therapists see that differently. In 1977, Petzold (398) wrote that one focus of his Integrative Movement Therapy was to "work in the correction and rehearsal of behaviour." Leibold (1986, 122) went even further: "In the case of deeper muscle groups that cannot be treated from the outside, the therapist uses other techniques to break through the muscle armour." Instead, gestalt therapy has always been about liberating the individual from societal pressures to conform that were learned and embodied in the family. So, normative (physical) adaptation cannot be a gestalt technique.

Every contact with novelty, each new experience and all creatively adaptive behaviour is physical. The body itself is forged by emotions: "When we repress tears, we achieve this by repressing the flexibility of the muscles around the eyes, which will stiffen so as not to respond to the tremor induced by the emotion that would make us cry" (Spagnuolo Lobb, 2015, 22). This again points to the close reciprocal relationship between the physical and the experienced body. It recognizes that our bodies are the product of expressed *and* repressed emotions. These embodied memories are highly relevant for the course of therapy. Therapeutic success is not built on mentalisation but on relevant experiences that are fundamentally physical. Based on Schmitz's self-proclaimed 'new phenomenology' however, a few gestalt therapists claim that there are two stages of development: personal regression plus distancing/ explication (cf. Zielke, 2017, 23). For neo-phenomenologists, explication means to "explain or unfurl something to oneself" (Matthies, 2013, 87) – *after* a regressive event. To me that is an aberration. Certainly, therapy involves experience *and* integration. But neither are those two separate phases nor are they equally impactful or relevant. In gestalt therapy, relevance is not conferred ex post – it is experienced and realised *during* aware contact. "Normally, the process of the gestalt completion (homeostasis) is taking place on the non-verbal, even unaware level" (F. Perls, 2019, 20). F. Perls et al. (1951/2013, 422) did not see post-contact as a merely conscious reflection, but as a "passage from aware contact to unaware assimilation". So, therapy is neither a sequence of events nor a rational digestive process at all, but a constantly flowing mix of thoughts, emotions, physical activities and felt body awareness.

For any change and growth to occur, it is much more important *how* an individual deals with contact than *what* the issues of the original conflict were. Healing comes through awareness of these processes in the here and now. Or, as Yontef put it, "When one is aware, one does not alienate aspects of one's existence; one is whole" (quoted in Hycner/ Jacobs, 1995, 61). This kind of awareness, including physical and affective processes, is central to the course of therapy because contact with otherness needs the physical and felt body. If the therapeutic goal is maximum awareness, then we – therapists and clients – necessarily direct our attention to the physical and phenomenal contact processes here, now and for-next. Gestalt therapists have always insisted that the *client's body* is an important means for awareness (cf. L. Perls, 1992, 151). The physical body enables or limits experiences and at the same time it 'tells' the aware therapist what a client is experiencing. In the original, personalistically oriented gestalt perspective, the focus often was on the therapist's ability to perceive the body language expressions of their clients and to use them to foster their awareness. Based on this outlook, the inclusion of body processes serves to understand the contact styles of clients. Gestalt therapists use their own awareness as a diagnostic tool. "Metzger states that an adequate diagnosis also means that we can understand aspects of the client that he himself is not aware of or does not yet understand …" (Wollants, 2012, 45). Colleagues from other therapeutic orientations have taken a similar approach (see Fromm et al., 1972, 144). However, a personalistic or organismic perspective does not explain how an intimate understanding between separate first-person-singulars is possible at all, as explained in chapter 2. So, with regard to content-related, i.e. meaning-related interpretations of body language including the "non-verbal micro-processes" (Staemmler, 2009, 73), caution has been advised. For personalistic therapists, physical phenomena only make sense in the subjective context of the person perceiving them. The process of 'meaning making' is seen as an individual's activity. So "comprehension is at least always necessary when it is a matter of human-created structures, objects, symbols – that is, the interpretation of a human world" (Jung, 2001, 10). In this respect, gestalt therapy has always been phenomenological *and* hermeneutic, and it has included at least two people: a client and a therapist.

For gestalt therapists, diagnosis and treatment are not separate processes. "In fact, the diagnosis is therapy, and the therapy is diagnosis" (Spagnuolo Lobb, 2013, 253). In the course of our work, we pay attention to embodied feelings and to physical expressions of our clients' contact styles. We register the "primary physiology (like breathing and digestion), upright posture and coordination, sensitivity and mobility, language, habits and customs, social manners and relationships, and everything else that we have learned and experienced during our lifetime" (L. Perls, 1992, 144). In gestalt therapy we do not focus on our clients' mental ideas about the world which are interspersed with introjects. Instead, the affective experiences of the clients are crucial. Contact, therapy's first reality, has always been a central tool for gestalt therapists. "The more sensually a contact process is experienced, the more likely it is to become a satiating experience" (Dreitzel, 2007, 63).

7.3 The relational turn of gestalt therapy has focused on contact between therapist and client

Yet, in therapy sessions there is a lot more going on than the personalistic perspective is able to illuminate. Therapists are not just individuals who collect information about their clients and make it available to them by experiential interventions. In the perspective of a *relationally turned gestalt therapy*, the 'inner' pathology of a person is no longer the centre of attention. In shifting from a monopersonal paradigm to a situational, relational paradigm, the gestalt-theoretical approach has revised its paradigm of pathology as based on intrapsychic conflict and defence to an interactive conception of psychopathology "in which mental disorders are defined as behaviour and not as a defect within the person" (Wollants, 2012, 37). Instead of diagnosing and treating an individual's disorders, dialogue became the centre of relational gestalt therapy. The interaction between client and therapist came to be seen as a theatre of contact archetypal for behaviour in the wider field. Laura Perls (1992, 132) had long pointed out the fundamental need for support. In a relational perspective, that was no longer about assisting another person's affective, emotional, and mental processes. The relationship between therapist and client itself became the object and essential lever of awareness or growth, since "the relation to the therapist is a real social situation" (PHG, 1951/2013, 406). Our clients' mode of contact employed during therapy became a source for experiments and novel experiences. Since clients (and therapists) show the same contact behaviour as in other relationships, the focus of relational gestalt therapy is neither a conflict between the individual and their environment nor a creative adaptation nor unfinished gestalts of an individual. In this view, therapy is mainly about the contact behaviour here, now, and for-next, plus the implied co-created meaning-making process 'between' client and therapist.

For a relational gestalt therapist, 'dysfunctional' behaviour happens in the here-and-now contact. Thus, it can be dealt with more directly and differently in therapy. To some extent relational ideas were already present at the foundation of gestalt therapy. Only now the idea was used in a new manner: "all that can be known is the experiencing of the two participants" (Hycner/Jacobs, 1995, 147), i.e. of client and therapist. In the *shared situation*, they create meaning together and define a "consensually determined reality" (ibid., 149). They co-create the situation. For relational gestalt therapists, change continues to evolve from awareness (not from consciousness) and the nature of therapeutic interaction is not merely *exemplary* for life outside. The shared situation is real, it is the here-and-now-for-next in which meaning is co-created. Seen this way, therapy is only one tract of a much larger field. Unlike classic analysts, relational gestalt therapists do not see themselves as situated beyond, outside or above therapeutic processes. They are deliberately and awarely in contact with their clients. They immerse themselves in the experiences of their clients; they communicate their perceptions and experiences both verbally and non-verbally (cf. Hycner/Jacobs, 1995, 141). In these processes, two individuals do not each create meaning for themselves and subsequently communicate it. They do not share internally pre-formed ways of seeing or experiencing. It is during the (non-)verbal communication process that meaning emerges from the first reality (cf. Wheeler, 1991, 311). In contact, the expansion of mutual awareness changes perceptions, structures of meaning, interpretations, views, attitudes, as well as behaviours of all participants. From a relational perspective, this is not an individual act, but a co-creation: the encounter of otherness by its very nature gives birth to novelty, changing both client and therapist. Implicitly (if not explicitly), relational gestalt therapy ended the idea of bracketing the therapist's world.

Based on relational gestalt therapy, the interaction between therapist and client is interpreted differently. What was seen as a mere diagnostic tool has turned into the key focus of therapeutic experimentation and experience. Against the ground of physical and experienced conditions, affordances, limitations and opportunities, individual aspects of the relationship between therapist and client become gestalt – or not. Through the joint exploration of their environmental field, including the unfinished stories that tie up energy and keep pushing for the repetition of older patterns of behaviour, therapists do not just gain information about their clients. Their presence influences the figure-forming processes and behaviours: "Attunement [to clients – LG] is an event of great therapeutic value in and of itself, as it is a central phenomenon in the process of recognising the client and contributing to the validation of their experience" (Francesetti, 2020, 51). Only new and relevant experiences change relational behaviour. A prerequisite for this is meaningful support during therapy. Therapists are to feel the other side, the patient's side of the relationship, "as a bodily touch to know how the patient feels it. *If the patient could do this, there would be no need of therapy and no relationship*" (Buber quoted in Hycner/Jacobs, 1995, 79). The availability of the therapist offers support. In contrast to Fritz Perls, Laura Perls (1992, 132) already emphasised the importance of support: "Contact is possible only to the extent that support for it is available." If clients do not experience sufficient non-verbal and verbal support, anxious excitement is mobilised and previously learnt self-protective behaviours are employed to 'survive' perceived threats. Without support, novelty cannot be experienced. In relational terms, the success of therapy depends on how and to what extent therapists and clients succeed in co-creating support through contact as a basis for experiencing novelty.

At the same time, the therapeutic situation involves (renewed) contact with frightening aspects of experience. Therapists start from what the patient brings in. Yet if they only follow where the patient leads, "then the patient will evade and run circles. Therefore, as soon as one notices a crucial resistance (according to one's conception), one 'hammers' at this" (PHG, 1951, 283). Clients are believed to avoid pain-inducing topics or experiences at all costs. More precisely both in Perls' personalistic and in later relational perspectives, it has been assumed that clients avoid change when old fears become virulent. Thus the problem continues to be seen located within the realm of one individual – either the client's mental and emotional processes or their contact-making. In either case emerging figures that trigger fear are warded off by a fearful monad. The appearance of such figures during therapy is seen as an indicator of the client's attempts to protect themselves from affective overload. But for gestalt therapists, contact always means encountering novelty. Without a crisis and without clients getting in touch with their fears, "there is no healing from the gestalt therapeutic point of view" (Dreitzel, 2004, 124). Strangely, this ambivalence is what brings clients to a therapist's office in the first place. While they are keen to avoid pain they are not looking for a mere confirmation of their long-established ways of experiencing and behaving. They are aware (to a certain extent) that this is precisely what would cause them further pain. So how much are we to actually 'hammer' at them?

Unlike in California in the late 1960s, gestalt clients are no longer expected to act out repressed affects or feelings. I share Dreitzel's (2004, 127) "reservations about an exclusively cathartic conception of therapy." The goal of gestalt therapy is expanded awareness, through a supported and meaningful experience called "safe emergency" (PHG, 1951/2013, 286 and 288; also Kepner, 2008, 83). Gestalt therapists have always believed that they must "learn to work with sympathy and at the same time with frustration. These two elements may seem incompatible, but the therapist's art is to fuse them into an effective tool. He must be cruel in order to be kind" (F. Perls, 1973, 106). For relational therapists it is the co-created awareness of both frightening *and* supporting aspects of the field, which mobilises the drive for experimental behaviour. In that view therapists are no longer tasked to enable another individual to bear their pain and hammer at them, but to provide a mode of contacting that allows for modulated arousal and contained anxiety. The relational aim of therapy is not a replacement of environmental support with some dormant ability within a client's ego. Instead, therapists need to be present as a whole person in the situation. We lend our flesh to our clients, as Francesetti (2019, 48) calls it. In this respect, we necessarily also use (respectful!) physical interactions, because physical contact, experienced as supportive, sustaining, and resonating is central to human survival and life (cf. Jurkstaite-Paceesiene et al., 2018, 267). This has never been truer than in times of crisis.

7.4 Relational gestalt therapy is still based on an individualistic outlook

The personalistic task of therapy is to "illuminate a dark corner in the patient's awareness" (L. Perls, 1992, 146). For relational therapists, their presence delivers the necessary support so they and their clients dare to explore the 'dark' corners of the field and co-create new meaning. Our clients can trust that they no longer have to face their feelings of shame, fear, abandonment or grief alone. Relational therapists are 'intimate witnesses' who restore "the resonant self-field, for the renewed or ongoing resolution of new self-experience, new creativity, and renewed growth" (Wheeler, 2000, 279). Such an intimate witness does not provide superficial placations. They perceive the fearful experience and support affective-emotional arousal, "which is to say, *hearing and acknowledging the reality and distress of her apprehensive feelings themselves*" (ibid., 288). This undoubtedly alters previous experiences of shameful isolation. Hence, therapists represent a new opportunity by affording new experiences and change.

From a relational perspective, Hycner and Jacobs (1995, 64–73) expand the therapeutic task to a) presence, b) genuine and unreserved communication, c) inclusion, and d) confirmation. The reason for this explicit sequence still lies in the clients' needs: "Consequently, at the heart of a dialogically oriented psychotherapy is the need for the client to be confirmed by the therapist" (ibid., 24, quoting a client). While gestalt's relational turn shifted our theoretical and practical awareness further towards the field, it did not change the underlying individualistic paradigm, however. Clients still appear needy or defective or defensive – only the locus of the problem has altered. Accordingly, an essential goal of therapy now is the relational re-nurturing of clients through wholesome contact. This is to compensate for the individual's needs that were hitherto unsatisfied. Such processes 'between' therapist and client are seen as a 'back-and-forth' (ibid., 20) between two individuals *in* the field. Accordingly, inclusion is conceived as "a concrete imagining of the reality of the other in oneself, while still retaining his or her self-identity" (ibid., 68). So the relational outlook, too, cannot solve the problem of intersubjectivity, as elaborated in chapter 2. With its relational turn, gestalt therapy has moved even further away from Freudian analysis. As therapists we are no longer demigods behind the couch, but the intimate witnesses of our clients as they seek "validation of his or her *real* self" (ibid., 125). Yet, when relational gestalt therapists draw on ideas about an 'original' authenticity and a supposed 'true being', they confirm gestalt's original individualistic foundation. Much like their predecessors, they aim to "preserve the autonomy and detachment of the therapist from the client" (Staemmler, 2009, 27). The first generation of gestalt therapists was firmly rooted in solid modernity defending suffering individuals from the onslaught of societal impositions. The relational generation often references 'postmodern' narratives. By and large however, their experiences are still rooted in their usually privileged lives within the first world's liquid modernity.

The essential progress of gestalt's relational turn is its focus on the co-created meaning-making processes. It is precisely through this change of perspective that "new possibilities for growth and change in the shared field of self and other people emerge" (Wheeler, 2000, 179). The basis of this orientation is an *implicit* realisation that awareness is not an achievement of autonomous individuals. Every experience of reality, every experiment and its support, as well as every behaviour beyond the therapy session, is co-created. As supporters, disturbers, providers of feedback, physical objects, experienced bodies and more, therapists are part of their client's field physically and experientially. In a personalistic perspective, change occurs when previously learnt patterns of behaviour are altered by the individual. That means both I- and personality functions are adjusted. In a relational view, change and growth come about through new meaning-making in the co-created process 'between' individuals. This shifts the locus of change, which unfortunately is a vague 'inter-esse' where individuals still appear as subjects *in* the field. But the process of 'inter'-action is by no means as mysterious as it is sometimes portrayed: "Vibrations arise between therapist and client that require the therapist's attentiveness. Something oscillates back and forth, responds to the other (response resonance) or common oscillations arise (synchronous resonance)" (Baer, 2012, 321f). This may be a neat phenomenological approximation, but it occults *how* the process actually takes place. What is missing is an understanding of the fundamental importance of real (not merely metaphorical) resonances as physical and felt field vectors. As long as individuals are seen as the first reality, essential processes remain in the shadows.

Relational gestalt therapists emphasise "that meaning is relational in nature and emerges from the mutual interaction of figure and ground, of the observer and the observed, of self and other, of client and therapist" (Van de Riet, 2001, 188). What at first appears to be a banal gestalt therapeutic statement implies serious consequences for clients and therapists. The creation of meaning is only conceivable in resonance, not as a process within an individual, or in some undefinable in-between. The necessary basis for co-creation is a lively reverberation of another 'I' – not a mere echo. Regarding the therapeutic process, Francesetti et al. have summarised the differences between personalistic and relational gestalt perspectives (2019, 12–14):

The **personal perspective (A)**:

- "*What is changing?* The person in front of us."
- "*How can the therapist support the change?*" The change is enabled by the therapist's interventions raising awareness in a safe emergency. Thus, the client acquires the ability to experiment with and experience new creative adjustments.
- "*What supports the therapist as the third party?*" The model of contact styles is employed for diagnostic purposes and change is mainly observed on the level of ego-functions, i.e. what clients learn to do differently.

The **dialogical or relational perspective (B)**:

- "*What is changing?* Our relationship with the person in front of us." Therapy provides real relational experiences of otherness and novelty.
- "*How can the therapist support the change?*" Change is enabled by an engaged and aware dialogue. As therapists we offer new ways of contacting to be experienced, experimented with and thus co-created. The change is mainly happening on the level of personality-function addressing the question of who we are for each other.
- "*What supports the therapist as the third party?*" Therapists rely on the principles of inclusion, confirmation, presence, and commitment to dialogue.

These differences have far-reaching implications for psychopathology (ibid.). In the classical personalistic outlook "*psychopathological symptoms* are seen as the original creative adjustment of the organism" although they have become rather dysfunctional. Based on a relational perspective "*psycho-pathological symptoms* are seen as an individual expression of a specific relational experience" which changes through new relational experiences.

As helpful as these ideas have been, this is where the concept of an intimate witness falls short. Based on the Cartesian paradigm, the proponents of relational gestalt therapy seem to be stuck in a diffuse 'in-between'. If we think of therapy primarily as a meeting of predefined personalities, each with pre-existing perspectives, behaviours, and so forth, we miss essential field forces. If, however, we see contact as the first reality, it is two poles of a field that meet. On this basis and influenced by the physical conditions, demands, limitations and opportunities, the processes of perception and resonance take place, which in turn influence the phenomenological field. Therefore, therapists are much more than just intimate witnesses. They are partners in creation. Spagnuolo Lobb (2020) calls that "the dance of reciprocity between therapist and client." Still, such a relational dance is not about give-and-take. It affords listening to and following the valences of the field's music as well as creating new melodies. A resonant 'dance', as I understand it, is neither just an individual nurturing another, nor an alliance 'between' persons. In my view therapy is not about effecting change *in* clients or *with* clients, but about situational awareness, growth, and changes *of* the field.

Chapter 8

In the middle of therapy, the field has its seat[1]

Contact is the first reality of any situation. Thus, it is key to field-centred gestalt therapy. The physical and experienced bodies of client *and* therapist are access points to the resonant field structure, because "the subject is the conscious and creative recipient of this suffering: the subject can feel pain. The subject can perceive suffering and express it creatively, but suffering arises at the contact boundary" (Francesetti et al., 2016, 60). Bocian (2019, 124), on the other hand, seems to insist on an individualistic outlook: "I do not believe, however, that something like 'a field' or 'a relationship' that suffers actually exists." Yes, human pain is individual. It is experienced as one's own pain. This reflects a sound phenomenological approach. And still the success of therapy depends on how we look at what is going on. People are the sensitive 'poles'. Their suffering signals that the field or something of that field is out of kilter. We should assume that suffering is located neither *inside* the individual nor *in* the field.

8.1 Centring on the field is a paradigmatic turn for gestalt therapy

Seeing suffering as a field phenomenon is not new for gestalt therapists: "Koehler says, 'the whole-process is determined by intrinsic properties of a whole situation'" (PHG, 1951/2013, 255). Based on their personalistic outlook, the founders of gestalt therapy insisted that there is *no* function of any animal that is definable except as a function of such a field. For them organic physiology, thoughts and emotions, objects, and persons, are abstractions that are only meaningful when referred back to interactions of the field. "The field as a whole tends to complete itself, to reach the simplest equilibrium possible for that level of field. [...] An organism preserves itself only by growing" (ibid., 372). More recent publications have attempted to formulate this view more stringently, stating that "the isolated individual does not exist" (Francesetti, 2019, 38). Following a *'personal perspective'* and the *'dialogical perspective'*, some propose a **field theory perspective** (Francesetti et al., 2019, 15–17):

DOI: 10.4324/9781003454809-9

- *"What is changing?"* The dynamics of the id of the situation. Client and therapist are seen as processes formed here-and-now by the flow of the situation. The whole of the situation is more than the sum of people who meet each other and it transcends the persons involved.
- *"How can the therapist support the change?"* At the centre of the therapeutic approach is the therapist's aesthetic experience of the embodied presence. Change happens mainly on the level of id-function, i.e. the embodied undifferentiated needs which are a function of the situation.
- *"What supports the therapist as the third party?"* One the one hand therapists are supported by the concept of the paradoxical theory of change and by a keen awareness of co-responsive processes involving physical reactions of the client and first-person-singular sensations of the therapist.

Differing from previous gestalt approaches these ideas also impact psychopathology (ibid., 16). Instead of a disease-oriented definition of fixed symptoms that are somehow part of an individual, pathology is defined as *psychopathological situations* where "the natural flow of the situation is blocked, or rather distorted in a specific way."

In principle, I believe the approach proposed by Francesetti and others is a fruitful reformulation of gestalt therapy, because factually and experientially, it is not the subjects that form the initial element of reality, but "relations and dynamic relationalities" (Rosa, 2019a, 68), i.e. contact. Yet, in many respects their field perspective is still stuck in individualism. The authors seem to think that felt bodies can be hijacked by atmospheres and fail to describe what the targeted flow of the situation actually is. Their view is presented as a mere addition to the organismic point of view (Francesetti, 2020, 43). At the very least that is underselling the point and missing the potential. Taking this field perspective further, a new turn emerges which I call *gestalt therapy of the field* or *field-centred gestalt therapy*. This could be a Copernican revolution as it puts all the physical and phenomenal aspects of the field at the centre. On that basis, therapy no longer revolves around individual organisms nor relational in-betweens but around the emerging contact. This in turn offers solutions to various theoretical and practical problems. Of course, it also raises new questions.

If one wanted to put it this way, the 'object of treatment' is "the whole of a concrete person and his concrete phenomenal environment" (Wollants, 2012, 45, with reference to Köhler) – i.e. the situation. This term encompasses "all that is in situ" (Sarah Fallon, Appendix, in Wollants, 2012, 122). Despite the need to reduce complexity during concrete therapeutic processes, such a gestalt therapeutic orientation remains holistic. The objects of therapy (if one wanted to call them that) are not organisms nor a vague relational 'in-between', but the real and the experienced environmental relationships of living people. Subjects are perceptive poles of situational fields. They are themselves permanently re-constituted by the changing field while their reactions alter the very field. The phenomenological as well as the physical body is a reality that is always affecting and affected by forces, vectors and valences. Although still largely founded on a personalistic basis, Laura Perls (1992, 94) already described this principle: "The contact functions, by way of specific organ or a specifically structured activity, take place against a background of organismic functions which are normally unaware and taken for granted." Where there is contact, there is a field and vice versa. This idea can be a source of anxiety or a source of change and growth – both for clients and therapists.

What happens in contact is much more than a mere 'showing of oneself'. If we started from an individualistic foundation, we would conceptualise contact more like a sales pitch at Vanity Fair. Resonant contact is entirely different from a marketable display of personality features: "*A dialogue is centred in neither person, yet originates on both.* It is the recognition, deep in my being, of the mysteriousness and value of the other person as a person, who exists independently of my needs" (Hycner/Jacobs, 1995, 92). While the second part of the quotation points to the fact that resonances are something fundamentally different from contact between subjects and objects, Hycner and Jacobs rightly focus on what constitutes the 'more'. In my view this is the field, which remains hidden both in the original individualistic-organismic gestalt therapy and in the individualistic-relational turn (see chapter 7). Based on a consistent field-centredness, the old question of precedence of either environmental field or individual turns out to be as wrongly posed as that of chicken and egg: "In the mechanistic mode experiments can be devised to study this question in a linear fashion. But the question as posed creates a false dichotomy that is more easily dealt with in field theory" (Yontef, 1993, 287). The living environment is an assemblage of holistic, structured, co-created fields. Based on real physical processes, resonating contact is the first reality, because this differentiates the field into the experience of 'I' and 'not-I'. In this view, the unity of the field remains intact; actions are seen as functions of the field. The field is a unifying concept, not eliminating such divisions as 'person' and 'situation', or 'figure' and 'ground', but "denoting them as provisional and relativistic" (cf. Parlett, 1997, 18). The differentiations are not absolute or fixed. They constitute aspects of field processes; they are interwoven, in flux and ever-changing.

By consistently centring our outlook on the field, the concept of resonance yields benefits for gestalt therapy both in theory and practice: "Resonance is thus the main source of therapeutic behaviour" (*Dictionary of Psychotherapy* definition, quoted by Rosa, 2019a, 286, footnote 271). This is not meant as a mere metaphor. Resonances are real and felt phenomena of the field, structured by vectors (or intentionalities) towards resonance. So far, we have made only limited use of these processes in gestalt therapy: "In humanistic experiential therapies, including gestalt therapy, resonance has been used as a central tool of self-disclosure, with the therapist sharing her own experience" (Francesetti, 2020, 54). Is that all there is to it? Is resonance just another diagnostic tool or a relational building bloc? Francesetti (2020, 54) himself hints at more. Resonance, he suggests, "is the most valuable sign of the field we constitute and of the issues circulating within it between client and therapist" (ibid.). Is resonance then just a pointer to something else, perhaps to what Jacobs (2017) calls "*Enduring Relational Themes* (ERTs)"? Francesetti's answer is a vital step, but it does not tap the full conceptual potential.

8.2 Gestalt therapy is about exploring the resonant field emerging from contact

A *gestalt therapy of the field* builds on both personal and relational gestalt therapy using the idea of a "co-regulation of the shared field" (Fogl in Wheeler, 2000, 139). Meaning is not created by internal mental or affective processes. Meaning is always co-created. When we look at therapy from a field-centred perspective, the exchange 'between' therapist and client becomes much more nuanced: "Therefore, the therapist's act of sensing/perceiving is not only *empathy*, an identification with the client's experience, but also *resonance*, a personal and sensitive reaction to the field in the presence of the client" (Spagnuolo Lobb, 2018, 63). When relational gestalt therapists are present in the situation, they are already modulating the field. The centre of attention is not on witnessing a client intimately but on the interaction, i.e. the emerging vectors and valences. Yet, when we talk about contact styles, gestalt therapists often assume that these are preformatted by past experiences stored in the memory banks of an individual. Patterns of perception and action certainly limit a person's behaviour because they are designed to avoid pain. If we look at the field in toto, however, we realise old and new, available and unavailable, aware and unaware vectors of change have always been present. Pain avoidance is but one type of vector with a particular kind of valence. There are also other vectors. Growth, for example, is not about learning something new. It is primarily about discovering options already field-present. "Moreover, resonance phenomena are not the mere repetition of past scenarios, but the way in which the quality of the field here and now takes a perceptible form" (Francesetti, 2020, 53). In individualistic terms, apart from inhibiting factors such as fear or shame, the unfulfilled intentionalities for resonance are also part of a situation. Hence, therapy can do more than nurture individuals, help close old gestalts or provide an opportunity for (re-)nurturing relational experiences. The client "brings a legacy that seeks to exist here and now in order to reach the other and be transformed" (ibid.). This idea goes ever so slightly beyond the insights of individualistic gestalt therapy.

Field contact is the first reality of and for our clients: "The situation precedes the interacting parts of the situation" (Wollants, 2012, 66). To a certain extent, gestalt therapy has always been based on field theory. However, by means of a *consistent* field-centredness, therapeutic processes become much clearer. Therapies – much like other encounters – are not meetings of two preformed selves *in* the field. Our clients do not simply haul their old baggage into our offices. The therapeutic situation is a new, common field emerging from its inception. Its conditions, affordances, limitations, and opportunities are shaped by the structures of two previously separated fields and the emerging co-created forces, vectors, and valences. Thus, experiences, as well as potentialities, are present in the ground even when the poles remain unaware of them. What is or will become 'I' and 'not-I' respectively is being thrashed out by therapists and clients. Marková and Berrios (2019, 129) correctly state that meaning is established through negotiation. In English, the word 'negotiation' encompasses the alignment of interests and conversation, as well as the passage of difficult stretches of road or sea, the overcoming of obstacles and the management of danger. An apt term, I think, because it is a joint process and by no means a simple one. Therapy can be seen as the mutual construction of meaning "where through the dialogical exchange, utterances are selectively expressed, suppressed, responded to, elaborated and so on – within the negotiation demanded by the specific interaction" (ibid., 131f). In this view, gestalt therapy is a journey full of difficulties, dangers, and drawbacks. But it is also filled with opportunities, occasions, and options. Reality is not an individual construct – neither by a therapist nor by a client. It is co-created by experiments and explorations of the field. It is in this shared situation that an understanding of reality co-emerges. Seen from a client's point of view, the physical and felt contact with a therapist's field constitutes novelty. By its mere presence, it alters the structure and processes of the client's situation. Change and growth happen through exploring and experimenting with this co-created field while newly emerging vectors also affect the rest of a client's field (and that of the therapist). The experience of the field itself consisting of impressions and expressions already *is* looking, feeling, smelling, tasting and chewing differently, i.e. an altered mode of contact. "The embodied experience of relational uncertainty is how we can potentially live creatively" (Desmond, 2018, 185). Perceiving and assimilating is a novelty, not a pointer to something else or a process after the fact.

Analogous to Wheeler's understanding of meaning-making, the sociologist Miller (2015, 4.2) writes about the concept of understanding:

"In the work of phenomenological philosophers, it refers to the recognition that we consider each other's actions and words not as physically caused, but as the product of a dialogical relationship where interpretation of each other's gestures becomes the basis of a common reality created in the moment of interaction".

Miller hits on an essential idea despite the inner contradiction of this quote between actions that are not supposed to be physically caused and the interpretation of (physical!) gestures of another person. Reality and any 'construct' of it is always *shared*, it is *communicated* experience of the (therapeutic) situation and a *negotiated* creation of meaning. This idea also implies that co-creation is not only about understanding each other mentally or empathically. It is a resonating self-actualisation of the field that "arises as a by-product of enhanced relational connectedness" (Hycner/Jacobs, 1995, 94). To be clear, in my view the autonomy of an 'authentic inner self' with its 'inherent needs' can no longer be the acme of gestalt therapy. Rather I see self-efficacy and connectedness as poles of one and the same process. Therapy in that sense is about establishing, strengthening, and supporting the middle ground. In a common situation, it is not one *or* the other 'I' that develops something new. Reverberating resonances creates novelty, thus changing the structures, processes, and poles of the field. The decisive factor is not to be found *within* any of the involved individuals nor *in between* them. Rather, the 'treasure', the hitherto undiscovered opportunities for growth lie buried in the field that is the common situation. Rosa (2019a, 215) aptly suggests that relations with reality "are never given per se, but are constantly articulated, reconstructed, negotiated and transformed in individual and cultural processes of interpretation." This occurs as a function of the rich field of human resonance and contact.

8.3 The consistent use of the field paradigm expands the practical use of the body in therapy

"Intersubjectivity theory makes a strong case for reliable affect attunement as the means whereby the affect integration necessary for self-development occurs" (Hycner/Jacobs, 1995, 135). Just like the original organismic view, relational perspectives are largely based on an individualistic paradigm, which constitutes its limitation. In that vein Kepner (2008, 69) wrote about gestalt therapeutic bodywork: "The therapist is faced with the task of helping the client make the message from the body intelligible, and [...] restore the gaps in the organism." He defines the task of therapists as helping other people to experience themselves and decipher their existential messages from disowned parts of self. In their relational perspective, Hycner and Jacobs (1995, 84) wrote, "Patients must be afforded the chance to 'meet' another person if they are going to know themselves." In a field-centred perspective, however, therapy is about exploring the common field and thereby changing that very field including its human poles. The 'mutual attunement' is seen as *'field tuning'*, a modulating process *of* the common field, i.e. contact. Of course this is not a mental, intellectual, or mystical process. It is "kinaesthetic resonating" (Desmond, 2018, 185).

On a physical level, field resonances are affective reactions. Perceptions of these processes by therapists and clients are often experienced as quite diffuse at least at first (cf. Francesetti, 2020, 52). Emotional resonances are not mere signals "that 'I am present with you, regardless of our differences'" (Coburn cited in Miller, 2015, 4.6). Resonance is the first-person-singular's back reflection (with their own voice) in, of and to the situation. Experientially, too, resonances are not what emanates from one individual to another, but a field force. Precisely because resonance phenomena initially appear rather shapeless, therapists take risks using them: "When a resonance emerges, the therapist inevitably risks putting it into circulation by bringing it into play in a retraumatizing way" (Yontef, 2005). But re-traumatisation is not caused by *cognizant* perceptions of field resonances. As impressive and expressive experiences, they have long been part *of* the field, whether they were mentally represented or not. Indeed, as therapists we can ignore certain vectors and valences, but we cannot avoid reacting to them because, on a visceral, corporeal level we have already resonated whether we approve or not. Our "awareness is an element that makes the difference" (Francesetti, 2019, 57) enabling us to raise situational awareness.

"In the patient's posture, his shoulder posture, I see a lack of excitement that seems like sadness. [...] It is as if I feel his inner process, which is marked by loss and grief, physically as heaviness and immobility" (Wegscheider, 2015, 13). In the first part of the quote, Wegscheider refers to impressions of clients' bodies as a diagnostic tool. But he goes on to mention a more far-reaching idea: as therapists we resonate with our own body. We 'catch' emotions from our clients. No matter how our clients behave, they influence us, our physical and psychological perceived status. We "cannot learn anything about the patient independently of his or her own person and of his or her own influence on his or her opposite" (Streek quoted in Staemmler, 2009, 71), because we are also first-person-singulars *of* the situation. Intersubjective experiences are no projecting or speculating activities. Rather, they are physical and experiential field resonances – either concordant or complementary. A consistent, field-centred perspective of therapy is essential in order to become aware of and use one's own physical-phenomenal resonances as a resource. A field-centred turn of gestalt therapy expands our awareness of clients *and* of ourselves as therapists. It might also help therapists avoid confluence and re-traumatisation.

The idea of using the physical perceptions and reactions of therapists for either diagnostic or relational purposes is not new. Often, however, practitioners of gestalt therapy only concern themselves with their clients' *ex*pressions and their own *im*pressions. Yet, there have also been more wide-ranging ideas: "The therapist, just like the artist, also acts out his feelings, using his psychological state as an instrument for therapy. [...] One could say that the therapist becomes a sounding board for everything that happens between him and the patient" (Polster, 1995, 31). Therapists, too, react holistically to whatever is happening here and now in the therapeutic situation. Laura Perls (1992, 99) might have had this in mind when she wrote:

"I had only to consult my own reactions to the patient's behaviour, my awareness of being belittled and imposed upon, the feeling of hostility that she provoked in me, to realise the specific pattern that the patient was acting out in this meeting as well as in any other contact situation."

Therapists are 'infected' by the emotions of their clients. Based on a similar perspective, Spagnuolo Lobb (2020) describes crucial questions that therapists could use to guide their awareness: "What do I feel in front of this person? What movement do I perceive in myself? What energy do I feel in the field?"

The living body is part of an ongoing interaction and provides information about the situation. "The body carries information that is not (or not yet) capable of being formulated verbally. It is the task of therapists to bring this knowing into the client's awareness" (Wollants, 2012, 80). This task was formulated by the Flemish gestalt therapist regarding the awareness processes of our clients' physical expressions. I think the same applies to our own resonance phenomena, because "sensation is the raw data of experience, the background from which we begin to organize our functioning" (Kepner, 2008, 92). For the success of gestalt therapy processes, our awareness of our own (re-)actions is as important as our perception of our clients' contact behaviour. However, without the underpinning of resonance theory on the one hand and the ideas of affective-emotional, physical, and experiential contagion on the other, such notions open the door to esoteric or metaphysical speculations. In my view field resonances can be described phenomenologically and scientifically. So can their affordances, opportunities, and limitations. They become fully comprehensible and usable when gestalt therapy is consistently centred on field structures, processes, vectors, valences, and poles.

"From the perspective of field theory, the therapist's presence, biases, and behaviour continually interact with the client and contribute to how the client perceives, interprets, and creates meaning" (Van de Riet, 2001, 189) In this respect, the verbal, non- or para-verbal expressions are not only diagnostically interesting. The physical and felt reactions of therapists subtly or openly influence the experience of clients in a shared situation. Laura Perls (1992, 118) wrote that "in the course of the therapy the patient learns to become aware of my reactions and expressions just as much (and sometimes more so!) as I am aware of his, even if not verbalized". This cannot be otherwise, because in a therapeutic field, the poles involved are in resonant contact. Contrary to what phenomenologists thought 100 years ago, therapists cannot 'bracket' their first-person-singular perspective, because they are part of reciprocal resonances and their contagion reactions are forces of the field long before they become aware of them. Therapists are always *of* the situation "because as a participating observer and part of the situation we can experience facets of his being that he bodies forth and are active in his life space, but of which he is not aware" (Wollants, 2012, 45). Against this background, we cannot be out of contact – nor can our clients. Based on personalistic notions, there were already different opinions about this. What the patient must learn "is to recognise sharply when he is no longer in contact, how he is not, and where and what the actuality now is, so he can continue contacting it" (PHG, 1951/2013, 465). Yet Laura Perls (1992, 144) wrote, "Contact is nothing one has, or is, or stays in or out of." Looking at it from a field-centred perspective, the poles co-modulate their behaviour resonating with the first reality of the field. The idea of 'no longer being in contact' makes no sense anymore. There are always vectors for resonance. The focus of therapy should be the changes, modes, and strength of contact, i.e. the valences.

Our involuntary and physical reactions spread throughout the field as contagion. They modify the joint situational field and influence its structure, processes, vectors, valences, and poles. These effects are by no means monodirectional but float back and forth. For example, if I feel disgust for a client that would not be something I consciously choose to feel. If I sense such a reaction, I might at first want to ignore it, fight it, suppress it, or put it off until the next supervision session. Yet in either case my embodied resonance has long been present in the situation (cf. Appel-Opper, 2010, 52). What we express impresses our clients. So, I can never put my physical-affective resonance in parentheses, i.e. I cannot exclude it from the field volitionally. As a physical and experienced pole of the field, I cannot help but be present. As a gestalt therapist, I do this mindfully and intentionally, to support the negotiation process within the common situation. For this I gladly use Francesetti's term, "lending one's flesh" (2019, 48). This is not a metaphor, "but a concrete and simple experience, which lies in feeling something that does not already belong to me, but which comes from the field from which I emerge" (ibid.). Being a resonating pole is significantly more (and for me far more meaningful and touching) than just being an intimate witness of somebody else's suffering.

In a *gestalt therapy of the field*, self and field are not differentiated into inner or outer realms, but the field is holistic and structured. In that sense I "conceive of the self as an agency that in some way encompasses the whole field" (Wheeler, 2000, 227f). The id of the situation, its conditions, demands, limitations and opportunities are fundamental to the differentiation process of 'I' and 'not-I', both in terms of physical and perceived *ex*pressions that are always also *im*pressions. What the poles of the field might perceive as atmospheres is based on environmental conditions, spatial constellations, and bodily reactions that we physically experience on and in our own bodies.

They are our resonances to forces, vectors, and valences of the field. To be able to use this therapeutically, we will have to go beyond the personalistic and relational paradigm on which gestalt therapy has rested thus far. Instead therapists "need to follow the hidden 'wisdom' of the situation" (Roubal, 2019, 80). Gestalt therapy has never just been about applying a set number of techniques. Through our way of making aware contact, our posture and our bodily resonance, gestalt therapists are a resource of the field. As Roubal (ibid., 85) puts it, "It is not so important what we do, but how we are with the client." The art of being thoroughly present in the therapeutic situation alters the situation. The change happens by engaging completely, i.e. in an undisguised, unvarnished, and overt manner with what we perceive even if only diffusely. We surrender to it (in a manner of speaking) and allow its effects to blossom. This bears fruit for the entire field.

8.4 Being with otherness and novelty includes existential, experimental, and experiential uncertainty

Based on a consistent field-centred outlook, therapists and clients pause, for example, not because they are at a loss – although they might feel that way on occasion. To explore the common field sensitively and thoroughly they need to stay even with dimly perceived vectors. "Resonance is a vibration corresponding to 'something' that is *present* and at the same time *neglected* in the phenomenal field [...]. Thus, the therapist does not dismiss the resonance, he lets it be with a sense of curiosity" (Francesetti, 2019, 58). What is felt at first only dimly will emerge as it is a vector of the field. Such an attitude shares strong similarities with 'negative capability' described by the Romantic poet Keats: "I mean *Negative Capability*, that is when a man is capable of being in uncertainties, Mysteries, doubts, without any irritable reaching after fact & reason" (quoted in Hebron, 2014, 12). Keats' literary term refers to a condition of uncertainty situated between everyday reality and the countless possibilities of its perception or interpretation. It describes a state of purposeful open-mindedness and attentiveness. The attitude and behaviour necessary are known as the middle mode. When dwelling in uncertainty awarely, the evolving field vectors evoke perceptions in the form of prefigurations. These are resonances that spread through the field. "With *Vorgestalten* the perceptive experience is diffuse, undifferentiated, and global. The figure has yet to stand out separately from the ground; something is there, but it is an unstable, confused and indefinite presence" (Francesetti, 2019, 39). Perception – at least initially – does not take place as a rational, structured cognitive process. What impresses us physically may take time to really dawn on us.

However, such diffuse experiences do not only occur at the initiation of therapy or at the beginning of a session. For therapists, these unspecified and often quite irritating resonances mark a first undifferentiated contact with novelty and otherness. The fuzziness of that experience is a field phenomenon. The conditions, demands, limitations and opportunities of the situation imbue and colour the nascent experience. Yet the field's poles are not fully aware of and have not ascribed meaning to said experience. Influenced by the 'New Phenomenology', Francesetti (2019, 43) calls the occurrence pathic, dramatic, expressive, or poignant. Seen through the lens of a field-centred approach, these processes become clearer. Fleeting impressions are felt resonances either to atmospheric constellations of objects or to the spreading of subject–subject contagion through the field. To call this 'Vorgestalten' is helpful insofar as it describes a way of perception and aware contact without conflating it with either confluence or consciousness. In the context of field-centred gestalt therapy, however, the focus is on real *and* experienced perceptual processes, not on vaguely wafting atmospheres.

People perceive other poles, as well as the structures, processes, vectors, and valences of the field, even if they are not able to conceptualise them. Based on gestalt therapy's contact process model, this is not surprising. In the first phase of the contact, the quality of otherness comes into awareness as pre-figuration; the situational aspects of 'I' (e.g. its needs) and 'not-I' start to become gestalt. Claid (2018, 164) describes this as "being with difference rather than assimilating difference into sameness". The affective or emotional content of a situation can be felt but can often not be precisely classified or verbalised – at least not yet. At the onset of contact, i.e. "at the origin of perception, subject and object have yet to become separate; their differentiation is a product of the perceptive process" (Francesetti, 2015, 9). The distinction between 'I' and 'not-I' is not yet clear, because gestalt formation has only just begun. We all experience that we are connected to our environment and separate from it at the same time. Nevertheless, individual gestalt therapists adhere to the idea that contact – with objects or other subjects – somehow happens like a touch at the contact boundary (cf. Matthies, 2013, 77). That would only make sense if one wants to replace core gestalt therapeutic concepts with neo-phenomenological metaphysics. Thinking in terms of a consistently field-centred gestalt therapy, the understanding of contact boundary as a quasi-epidermis of the 'I' needs clarification. Gestalt therapy has always understood the contact boundary as a term for ongoing field processes consisting of demarcation from and connection with 'I' and 'not-I'. A key element of that boundary is not its delimiting function but its permeability because in "the course of this process, the organism changes its own structure" (Fuhr et al., 2001, 371). The boundary is perhaps where the perception of contact begins, but it is not the event's location nor an endpoint. Contact affects *all* aspects of the field. Perhaps Miriam and Erving Polster (1974, 101) had something similar in mind when they wrote: "Contact is in any case not compatible with remaining unchanged." When two people are in resonant contact, it is not only one gestalt formation that changes. The physical and perceptual ground, i.e. the common field structure is altered by the encounter of otherness and novelty. It is precisely these limiting and simultaneously catalysing conditions that give rise to new affordances and thus to new possibilities. Regarding the boundary, Kepner (2008, 166) has stated, that contact "involves some kind of exchange. In contact we take something across our self-boundary and render it into some form that is usable for our growth. We not only bring the environment up close, but into our self." I understand resonant contact as the self-frequency response of a field's pole (a person) by means of their own vibrancy. This applies reciprocally to all poles of the field. In this perspective, contact is a field phenomenon that does not happen at some boundary *in* the field. Boundary is a process function of the field not a location. Fore-contact, the initial encounter with novelty and otherness is just one phase of a broader process.

At the same time, an intentional openness and attentiveness as well as the ability to remain in the midst of an evolving field is highly important for gestalt therapists (cf. Robine, 2019, 175; also Robine, 1996 and Amendt-Lyon, 2019, 175). The pre-verbal awareness of the shifting vectors and valences during contact opens up new possibilities. "Aesthetic relational knowledge is the instrument through which the therapist resonates with the client during the session, as well as the lens through which he looks at the client's vitality"(Spagnuolo Lobb, 2018, 63). What the Italian gestalt therapist calls aesthetic knowledge is, in my view, nothing other than 'negative capability', the ability to maintain a position in the middle of the field. This is what I refer to as multiple, field-present, resonant, body-mimetic micro-processes. This intuitive abidance within indistinct pre-figurations is based on a holistic but as yet indistinct perception of the situation. These physical and phenomenal resonances always consist of both *im*pression and communicative *ex*pressions.

Based on a field-centred understanding of gestalt therapy, the concept of awareness and the tasks of therapists expand. Therapeutic awareness (at least initially) remains at an edge, without stepping into either direction. Derived from the Latin word limen, meaning 'a threshold', liminality describes a quality of ambiguity or even disorientation. This typically occurs in the middle stage of a rite of passage, when participants no longer hold their pre-ritual status but have not yet completed the transition to the status they will later hold. In that sense, therapists remain at the threshold. Their liminal occupation of the middle ground does not refer to a location or an abstract in-between. As a situationally anchored person, I am constantly reacting to atmospherically charged constellations of objects, and/or I resonate with subjective contagion. Gestalt formation begins with physical and phenomenal contact anchored in the situation. Liminal pre-figurations are transitional phenomena of sensing structures, processes, other poles, forces, objects, vectors, and valences of the field. Negative capability, liminality and aesthetical knowledge all reference the ability to remain in resonance and to experience gestalt formation rather than interfering with it, falling into it (confluence), mentalising or reflecting on it. This understanding of pre-figures enlarges our understanding of the field.

Based on a liminal sensing, field-centred gestalt therapy fosters further possibilities. An integral part of therapy is the (re)negotiation of contact styles. Here physical processes are basal. Attending to real and felt body resonances is not a simple diagnostic tool but an immediate and new experience in a safe emergency. Only practical action that is physically im- and expressed affects engagement and affords development. Starting from a field-centred paradigm, I define resonances as a key structural element of the field. This is based on multiple, field-present, resonant, body-mimetic micro-processes. The Czech gestalt therapist Roubal (2019, 74) comes close to this when he writes: "a dialogue with a depressed person immediately starts to slow down, time seems to crawl, and heaviness and tiredness falls on people around. The relational field organises itself in a depressed way". The "client and the therapist are functions of the depressed situation" (ibid., 72), i.e. all involved persons "are experiencing symptoms of depression themselves. They perceive a loss of ability to think clearly and to concentrate. On a bodily level, they feel stiffness, heaviness, weakness, and exhaustion" (ibid., 73). Furthermore, Roubal's descriptions illustrate that the felt phenomena can be observed and measured. With explicit reference to Hatfield (1994), he mentions a direct pairing or matching of the bodies of self and other. Synchronisation of gestures, postures or movements, for example, are observable physical events. When we define field phenomena as multiple, field-present, resonant, body-mimetic micro-processes, events become understandable. Contagious resonances are a "direct and unconscious feedback loop" that does not require "mental inferences" (Staemmler, 2009, 98). In field-centred gestalt therapy, we deal with vectors and valences of depressive or obsessive or fearful or shamed, etc., fields. We can approach these phenomena both from a phenomenological as well as an observable perspective.

8.5 Gestalt therapy should focus on the field/ground and resonating contagion effects

The actual field is structured regarding impressions, expressions and experiences of both therapist and client. When a situation is characterised by depressive vectors and valences for example, they dampen or mute resonating contact. People then become aware of a gloomy or lifeless atmosphere because the 'depressed field' lacks resonances. Multiple, field-present, resonant, body-mimetic micro-processes naturally cause the poles of a field to be in contact with each other long before they are aware of it. Human mimicry forms a unity of impression, experience, and expression. As intuition, hunches, or moods, it affects all poles in the situation. In a fraction of a second, we decide whether to mimic another person's facial expressions and respond to the physical expression either in a concordant or complementary way. To support our clients, a concordant reaction is often most helpful. Still, in order to create a safe emergency, spontaneous complementary resonances can also be valuable parts of the contact process. Either way, our spontaneous reactions affect the situation. They can be a beneficial part of the therapeutic process: "In gestalt-therapeutic practice, both my imitation of the body actions, gestures and facial expressions of the client and his seeing me mirroring these actions, gestures and expressions have a critical value" (Wollants, 2012, 79).

Of course, the physically experienced resonances of therapists are in turn perceived by clients as subtle communication (cf. Appel-Opper, 2010, 51). A therapist's body is necessarily part of the situation so we cannot stay out of the situational contact. *How* we use this is crucial. Contagion phenomena of therapists are interventions, irrespective of whether we are aware of them or not. If we see bodywork only as a diagnostic tool or as relational support for our clients, we are already distancing ourselves from the co-created situation. Thus we doctor our mode of contact, avoiding being fully present. Starting from an organismic- or relational-individualistic approach, we miss opportunities. Resonating contact is a field's first reality – also during therapy. Therefore, a negotiated modulation of effects is not only a method that can be applied. Multiple, body-mimetic micro-processes take place all the time. Hence, the focus is on modulating both figure formation and the ground, including the 'ids' of the field. This necessarily includes ways of managing affective arousal using options that are available.

"Field conditions of increasing activation and threat erode our capacity for relational contact and privilege bodily and behavioural responses that are geared more for survival than contact" (Kepner, 2016, 19). The object of therapy can no longer be to increase the wave of a client's excitation or to ask clients to act out their unbridled desires. In his lecture at the AAGT/EAGT conference in Taormina in 2016, Kepner clearly pointed out that simply increasing arousal is not at all useful. Unlike in Fritz Perls' time, growth is no longer about expressing some 'inner' unlived needs that are emotionally charged. Rather, Kepner (ibid., 14) suggests, the *shared* resonant behaviour during therapy sessions varies between "play", "engaged", and "recoup". This may or may not take the form of the familiar gestalt cycle. Again, I would like to stress that it is essential to remain in the liminal *middle* mode attempting to use the modulating forces of the emerging field to influence the self-same field as well as the ongoing figure formation.

Because of a field's vectors and valences towards resonance, the (therapeutic) field arises at the moment of first contact. "When therapist and client meet for the first time, consciously or unconsciously the capacity for compassion, sympathy, the possibility of intercorporeality is tested" (Baer, 2012, 300). What Baer nebulously calls 'intercorporeality' in essence is resonance. He rightly points out that resonances occur right from the start. However, that is not a phenomenon restricted to the very first encounter between individuals. It is a process that occurs all through therapy, whenever there is contact with novelty and otherness. Based on field-resonant processes, clients and therapists create and negotiate new meaning all along. They explore a field already altered by their mutual presence. Regarding his ideas of resonance, Miller (2015, 8.8) concludes, "In this respect, it is worth pointing out that in considering resonance as a social phenomenon we should consider the impact, and indeed the value of dissonance, and the process of having to come to terms with 'the unsettling'". What he refers to as 'unsettling' I would call complementary body-mimetic processes. Successful therapy requires physical and experiential resonance for all stripes, i.e. awareness and resonance for:

- the forces that shape relationships and that are effective aspects of the field (albeit often only diffusely perceptible), with the relevant conditions, demands, limitations and opportunities they include,
- figure-formations based on multiple, body-mimetic, affective-emotional processes, and
- the possibilities of the ground, the intentionalities that are new or have hitherto lain dormant in the field.

"There is no completion of unfinished physiological situations without, ultimately, new environment material for assimilation" (PHG, 1951/2013, 406). Based on modern individualism, the fundamental meaning of resonance remains unclear. The focus is only on individual needs, unfinished experiences, and new skills. Zinker (1977, 93) formulated the therapy goal accordingly: "Every person should be capable of becoming fully aware of and acting upon his needs." For him, it was about the individual autonomy of individuals vis-à-vis restrictive circumstances *in* the field, i.e. the social constrictions of previous, rigid modern times. Accordingly, the therapist structures, forms, and steers the process of figure formation generated by the relationship between themselves and their client. In this view, therapists are experts who help other less fortunate individuals. But Zinker (ibid., 17) also indicates ideas that go beyond personalistic individualism: "The creative therapist sees the client in his completeness", i.e. with their environmental references. From the perspective of field-centred gestalt therapy, it is no longer about nudging, nettling or needling individuals towards change: "The therapist is no longer seen to work on the client but, rather, seeks to modulate the field co-created together with the client through his own presence" (Francesetti, 2015, 7). Hence, therapy is also not only about the skilful application of methods or interventions. Therapists tweak the situation by their presence and their contagious resonances. They enlarge and enrich the conditions, demands, limitations and opportunities of the joint field.

Regarding an organism, Goldstein (1934/1995, 173) stated, "*Any change in one locality is accompanied by a change in other localities.*" This is equally true for therapeutic fields. From the point of view of a field-centred gestalt therapy, the presence and behaviour of therapists modulate the field *as a whole*, since structures, processes, vectors and valences change. The American gestalt therapist Robert Resnick (2019, 81) points out, "As any part of the situation changes – the person, the environment, the larger field, etc. – what's *due* the situation may likely change too." The expression 'what's *due* the situation' Resinck takes from Laura Perls. This is quite similar to what Wollant called the 'id' of the situation. The presence of new poles as well as new 'atmospheric' factors restructure the composition of the field and thus pose new affordances.

Gestalt therapy usually focuses on *how* gestalt formation takes place: "'Figure' is the focus of interest – an object, pattern, etc. – with 'ground' the setting or context" (PHG, 1951/2013, 25). Yet at any given moment, the ground furnishes a multitude of possibilities because "the same ground may, with differing interests and shifts of attention, give rise to different figures" (ibid.). The interplay between figure and ground is dynamic and changeable. Emerging figures may include affective reactions, perceptive patterns, emotions, opinions, points of view, values, attitudes, and more. The focus of attention in personalistic- and relational-individualistic therapy is on unfinished 'gestalten', i.e. experiences, happenings and stories of the client that have not (yet) been completed and therefore impede the current cycle of figure formation. Past creative adaptations gave rise to contact styles that are maintained here and now, even when they are experienced as burdensome, painful, or dysfunctional. If, on the other hand, I start from a field-centred approach, i.e. when I focus on the physical-phenomenal situation that is characterised by contact, therapy is no longer just about the foreground (the gestalt formations). Rather, the entire ground, with all its conditions, limitations, and opportunities comes into view. Under the heading "from the Support of the Figure to the Support of the Background", Spagnuolo Lobb (2013, 152f) suggests shifting the focus of the therapeutic work because uncertainty, unpredictability, and variability of the ground experience are key characteristics of liquid modernity. Volatile markets demand malleable I-, id-, and personality functions. Geuter (2015, 171) describes a 'normal' learning or development process: "Memories are coupled to new states, to a new experience, when they are recalled, discussed and relived in a different bodily-emotional-motivational condition." However, when knowledge, memories, skills, etc., rapidly lose their exchange value on shifting markets, the ground itself is massively disrupted and becomes unstable because of alienation. People feel a constant 'atmosphere' of unsafe emergency and a permanent crisis.

In such conditions, therapy should not be only about supporting an individually avoided figure formation against social pressures. In more and more cases therapy needs to stabilise the experience of self. Alienation has become a protracted personal experience. Hyper-individualistic markets force individuals to sell themselves and maintain both a fluid gestalt-formation and an equally shifting ground that does not mortgage their future. At the same time, self-entrepreneurs are asked to be recognisable brands, i.e. fixed 'gestalten'. Referencing therapeutic work with adolescents and young adults, Spagnuolo Lobb (2013, 147) specifies: "These young people must be provided with strong arms that can contain and relax the terrible stress they feel at having to live without the nurturing other, in an agonizing solitude in which everything is a demand for performance." Generally, she describes therapy as a possibility to experience field-changing resonances, *"resensitize the body,* and to give tools of *horizontal relational support"* (ibid., 33). Gestalt therapy is not a repair shop for defective 'products'. It provides human beings with opportunities to experiment with forms of contact not limited by the permanent assessment of exchange value.

8.6 Gestalt therapy should essentially be concerned with the fertile field

When we place the situational field at the centre of gestalt therapy – both in theory and in practice – another point becomes clear or at least clearer: awareness includes, at least potentially, the whole field as a horizon of possible forms. Figure formation is impossible without a ground that is distinct from it. "Field theory already implies the existence of a ground that gives meaning to the figure. In different situations, different figures can emerge from the background, anchoring the respective relation and giving it meaning" (Francesetti et al., 2016, 63). Under the conditions of liquid modernity, when markets demand that both ground and figure remain pliable, working the ground can no longer be taken for granted. However, it is important to not just shift to another object and remain fixed on deficits and deficiencies. The field is always more fertile and more colourful than current gestalt formations suggest. The ground offers more diverse possibilities than individuals suspect or can use at any given moment. The joint therapeutic field contains not only different but often contradictory demands and allows for diverse and divergent perspectives, feelings, or attitudes. Clients can experience anger, sadness, and relief at the same time. They can love and hate a counterpart or be simultaneously angry with them because different vectors and valences are present. In any situation we are only aware of a fraction of this potential: "In the ego-stage of creative adjustment the self identifies parts of the field as its own and alienates other parts as not its own" (PHG, 1951/2013, 447). We should also apply this to ourselves as therapists. We, too, are only ever aware of sections of the joint therapeutic field. What we perceive and what we orient ourselves towards could be decisive points for co-development – it could also be quite useless. This is not only because the situation is different for therapists than for the clients, but because the field itself – every field – offers so many more possibilities and affordances than can be perceived or lived in the here, now, and for-next.

Due to our resonances, the field as it has previously existed for our client changes. Together we are in contact with novelty and otherness. The common field begets new impressions, expressions, and new experiences, in short: new gestalt formations. So, we do not explore a pre-existing client field or two fields and their in-between. The co-created situation substantially expands and alters the real and experiential field as well as connected sub-fields. "It is *support from the whole field that energizes us and makes change possible*; it is the *absence or constriction of new support that makes an old pattern, an old organisation of the field, persist and resist change*" (Wheeler, 2000, 218). Organismically, that might be understood as model learning or as a transfer of skills, abilities, and knowledge. But in fact, many of our successes in therapy come from an unrestricted unfolding of the first reality. "Any behaviour or other change within a psychological field [... is ...] solely dependent on the psychological field *at that time*" (Lewin, quoted in Wengraf, 2016, 16). The awareness of therapists and clients, their readiness for a supported experience of existential crises, as well as the relational freedom for experimental behaviour are directly dependent on the structure of the co-created field, especially its supportive vectors and valences. In this sense, therapists expand the field of their clients not only by providing safety in experience (as an antidote to the experienced excitations). At the same time our presence provides stimuli and new possibilities. Because we are in contact, our behaviour, the setting, the constellated atmosphere, and other factors afford alternative perceptions, experiences, im- and expressions. Due to such new circumstances, the ground itself has changed, making new gestalt formations possible.

"We know that the human organism has both physiological and psychological needs for contact in order to stay alive" (Schnee, 2018, 33). In field-centred terms: since contact is the first reality, resonance is a fundamental vector/intentionality, both physically and phenomenally. Eugene T. Gendlin, the founder of focusing, summarised, "I change as I speak and think and feel, because your reactions are part of my experience at every moment" (quoted in Staemmler, 2009, 93). When I take this as my starting point, field modulation through physical and experienced resonance becomes a central point of therapy. Creative adaptations (or better: field modulations) take place not only in situations that our clients experience as painful or restricting. Regarding shame, Josta Bernstädt (2017, 15) writes, "Internalised shame has thus arisen in relation to a vis-à-vis (intersubjectively) and was usually conveyed non-verbally in early childhood." It was the result of non-resonating relations. When children are shamed, 'healing' can come from a field expanded and enriched by therapy. Field-modifying resonances are decisive game-changers because "we cannot be part of a field in which shame is evoked with awareness for another person, without testing and being thrown back on our own capacity to process and bear our own experiences of shame" (Wheeler, 2000, 259). The vectors and valences of shame are contagious. For the poles, they are embodied feelings, experiences, impressions, and expressions. The same applies to other feelings such as pain, sadness, depression, anger, joy, pleasure, etc. Because of physical and phenomenal contagion processes, therapists cannot reject contacting shame or any other feeling. However, like all other people, we can ignore, repress, or ward off our reactions. We can refuse to be aware of our resonances or we can nurture our own narcissistic tendencies by cajoling our clients to echo us. Our clients' figure formation is then influenced by the same old vectors of 'silent' communication once again. Only when therapist and client together become aware of the supporting and 'safe' valences that are present, the influence of previous vectors can be modified.

The setting of therapy, including our resonant presence, allows our clients to negotiate new conditions, demands, limitations and opportunities. This is substantially different from a merely "deconstructive dialogue" (Wheeler, 2000, 131). Field-centred gestalt therapy is neither about deconstruction nor about model learning as suggested by Rosa (2019a, 280f): a subject's expectation of self-efficacy grows, he writes, "when a subject observes other (similar) individuals", who are relevant to the resonance process, "successfully accomplishing a task". A gestalt therapy of the field is about the co-creation of new meaning by exploring, restoring, and modulating the field, because the resonances of the common field immediately provide new conditions and demands for awareness and contact behaviour. Thus, a field-centred gestalt therapy confirms basic ideas of both the personalistic and relational orientation. At the same time, it shifts the object of therapy because visualising therapy as the meeting of two individuals confirms the demands of liquid modern markets. Therapists and clients enliven the rich field, 'growing' new figures. Together, they negotiate, explore, and experiment with the field. Awareness of as many aspects of the fertile field as possible paradoxically brings about change. Hence, the experience of self and self-efficacy is the result of complex negotiations with otherness including identifications and delineations.

Note

1   *Adapted sentence by Copernicus, N. (1543): De revolutionibus orbium coelestium, quoted after:* www.aphorismen.de.

Chapter 9

My gestalt of therapy

The aftermath of contact is accomplished growth[1]

Therapists as well as practitioners of other professions have taken the whole field into consideration: "A holistic view of the human being starts from the original unity of organism and environment" (Scheurle, 2013, 79). As gestalt therapists, we look at the entire co-created situation during therapy sessions and at our clients' lives outside our premises. Wollants (2012, 95) summed it up when he wrote, "Starting from the *total* situation, we have to take into account all the forces that influence the person's situation here and now." People are not single entities and contact is their first reality. Based on the social conditions, demands, limitations and opportunities of liquid modernity described in chapter 1, people are ever more alienated from each other. Impersonal market rules push them to see each other's personalities as commodities and assess each other's exchange value. As that is an essential part of our clients' life experience, alienation should be an integral part of gestalt therapy theory and practice. Alienation is existential and experiential and it is phenomenologically describable:

- people around me only react to such signals, "which I myself do not care about at all" (Henning, 2015, 122),
- people who are important to me do not agree with how I see myself or wish me to be different, and
- I live in a context "in which things are considered important that are unimportant to myself" (ibid.).

As existentialists have argued for some time, it is only through active engagement with one's environment that humans create their 'being'. "Labour not only produces commodities, but also the worker" (K. Marx, quoted in Henning, 2015, 118). People are fundamentally free to decide and act. At the same time, they are part of situations, including physical 'ids'. Their "given space of possibilities" (Henning, 2015, 199) presents demands, limitations, and opportunities. What makes people tick is their striving for self-determination and growth. At the same time, they can only

DOI: 10.4324/9781003454809-10

realise their aspirations through attachment, belonging and resonance. Based on the ideology of hyper-individualism, the idea of independence, however, becomes an obsession and human contact is turned into a product. "Nordic Cuddle Therapy" (Samadder, 2019) touted in the UK and the US, offers to square that circle. Intimacy is to be an experience purchased on the market. However, as a marketed item, closeness cannot strengthen the I-, id- or personality-functions because it is neither mutual nor does it engage with forces present in the real-life field of customers. It is a kind of Ersatz therapy, much like positive thinking, or a Biedermeier-like retreat into the wisdom of the cosmos (e.g. Lindau, 2019). It reveals the extent of human isolation and alienation in liquid modernity and does nothing to alleviate it.

9.1 Growth should be the central focus of gestalt therapy

As an antidote to the 'silent' affordances of market conformity, resonant contact is the central tenet of any *field-centred therapy*. "Resonance means reinforcement", Scheurle (2017, 40) claims. However, what is it we reinforce with our therapeutic resonances? Perls, Hefferline and Goodman commenced from a focus on interest with ground as its setting (PHG, 1951/2013, 25). Thus, the first element of therapy should be our clients' mode and quality of contact with us – the nourishing value, if you will. Without sustenance from the environmental field, i.e. without contact with otherness, the self remains hungry. Or to put it another way, due to alienation from certain forces of the field, development and growth stagnate. Because of the dominant affordances of liquid markets, the field will even regress. In gestalt-therapeutic processes, contact with and awareness of novelty is central. This includes the co-creation of experiences in therapy that are meaningful beyond the practice room. Growth, this life-sustaining integration of otherness, can only happen with another person resonating: "When we feel known and know others, our experiences are more certain, in what Schulz termed the 'vivid presence'" (Miller, 2015, 3.6). Consequently, it is not about some I–Thou in-between in which individuals remain singular entities brushing up against each other's boundaries. More pointedly, what walks through the doors of our offices is not an individual but a physically embodied field that begins to change the moment we become a novel pole of it. In contact, client and therapist co-create and alter their fields. The point of therapy is not to re-establish a new equilibrium after contact but to provide contact with novelty fostering growth. Therapy (and contact in general) should be about "we relationships" (ibid., 3.8). This not only grounds clients – and therapists, by the way. It also counters the desensitising forces of liquid society: "*Real therapy,* however, *is* not adjustment to society alone, *but the integration of 'self-actualisation', and identification with the sane needs of society, and with the cosmos* (laws of nature)" (F. Perls et al., 2019, 48). Rephrased in field-centred terms: therapy should lead to or strengthen the identification with the 'sane' Ids of society.

"The true purpose of man [...] is the highest and most proportionate formation of his powers into a whole" (Humboldt quoted in Henning, 2015, 71). Yet all too often I get the impression that publications about therapy only focus on the difficulties, deficits, and disorders of our clients: "Gestalt therapy treats disorders of this life process" (Blankertz/ Doubrawa, 2005, 179). Even field-oriented gestalt therapists all too often deem the problems of our clients more important than their achievements and strengths (cf. Francesetti et al., 2016, 65). Based on his analytical training, Fritz Perls, Hefferline and Goodman summed up the core of their (personalistic) approach: "Psychoanalysis has stressed recovery of awareness of what is repressed – that is, the blocked impulse. We, on the other hand, emphasize recovery of awareness of the blocking, the feeling that one is doing and how one is doing it" (PHG, 1951/2013, 148). As gestalt therapists, we focus on the *how* (the processes) and not so much on the *what* of a situation (the content). Based on a personalistic gestalt outlook, we assist our clients in becoming aware of how they themselves maintain the blockages and pain. An in-depth awareness of how their experience unfolds is meant to complete the original intentionality and fulfil an unachieved need. Based on a *field-centred approach* our focus shifts. Of course, our clients' fields and the perceptions thereof are saturated with pain and suffering. Why else would they seek us out? But that is not all that is present. Long before they set foot in our office, the field was so much more fertile and richer. Ultimately, when clients come to us, they intend to alter disabling forces and vectors. They also want to strengthen those pointing towards growth.

For gestalt therapists it has long been clear: "Neurotic behaviours are creative adjustments of a field in which there are repressions" (PHG, 1951/ 2013, 447). Bowman (2019, 63) elaborates: "Gestalt therapy has evolved from the idea of 'resistance' through 'interruptions of contact', 'contact disturbances', 'boundary disturbances', or 'boundary processes' to a more relational and field model of creative adjustments." What clients suffer from are the unhelpful consequences of their creative adjustment processes. In other words, these gestalts were adjustments to previous field factors that were (and often still are) characterised by pressure, fear, shame, etc. So any neurotic field is always ambivalent because "the symptom is both an expression of vitality and a 'defence' against vitality" (PHG, 1951/2013, 284). The founding document of gestalt therapy already made that clear. What others had interpreted as symptoms of illnesses is an attempted solution to an unendurable problem. In the beginning, there was a real and/or perceived, insoluble conflict between impulses to act and threatening field forces that stifled momentum. But instead of trusting in our clients' gestalt formation, the therapeutic attention is all too often only on the hindering aspects, the so-called resistance: for the patient "to walk in at all is partly a 'defence' against his own creative adjustment, a resistance against his own growth, as well as a vital cry for help" (ibid., 283). Exactly! Clients are afraid of change and *at the same time* their presence in therapy expresses their yearning. In field-centred terms, as vectors for growth are already present, they trigger experiments, experiences, and awareness, i.e. the wish to contact novelty. Key questions for therapists are then: Which field forces do we primarily resonate with? How can we resonate with our clients' yearnings if we focus so much on individual or relational neurotic behaviour?

Supposedly our clients are caught in an 'inner' conflict between needs-fulfilling intentions and forces that restrict these very actions. Although gestalt therapists (should) have this in mind during some sessions, at times it sounds more as if they are driven to get their clients to do something: "the strategy is always to keep a steady gentle pressure toward the direct and responsible I–Thou orientation, keeping the focus on awareness of the difficulties the patients experience in doing this" (Enright in Stephenson, 1975, 25). Of course Enright adds that therapists should help clients to *find their own way* through these difficulties, but there is that orientation towards (subtle) pressure which I find unhelpful. Rather, such self-aggrandising attitudes should urgently be dealt with, probably in the context of supervision. In today's hyper-individualistic environment, the question is: How can clients and therapists deal with the forces of the field that oscillate between desire and dread? How can we attend to the field in its entirety, using our visceral resonances in an aware manner? "In the present lies hidden what can *become*" (Friedman quoted in Hycner/Jacobs, 1995, 72). Based on a field-centred outlook, it is time to refocus our therapeutic efforts towards the *field forces for growth*.

Gestalt therapy of the field involves an unshakeable belief in the possibilities of the field. This needs to be grounded in *certainty* about the first reality of any field: "*It is the intentionality of contact implicit in the field that determines the meaning of the experiences, not the inner needs of the single individuals*" (Spagnuolo Lobb, 2013, 169). In this respect, an essential question throughout therapy is: Which field vectors sustain creative behaviour and which induce restricting actions? What divergent vectors are behind our clients' habits? In my opinion, vectors for growth should be the central point of orientation for therapeutic processes because "the co-creation of the therapeutic experience is motivated – supported and directed – by an intentionality, which for the gestalt approach is always an intentionality of contact with the other" (ibid., 33). The resonances of gestalt therapists should mainly be oriented towards these expanding vectors and valences, since they represent important conditions, demands, and – most importantly – opportunities: "The therapeutic intervention is focused on supporting that intentionality of contact" (ibid., 33), i.e. on encountering novelty and otherness awarely. Resonance with otherness induces growth.

9.2 Intentionalities are the felt field markers of growth

When we gestalt therapists focus mainly on the *growth vectors of the field*, our attitude shifts. "I believe that the therapeutic action must support what the patient already is able to do, rather than modify what does not work" (ibid., 49). Together with our clients, we focus on the forces fostering growth. Since these are usually not the vectors that are part of the client's currently aware gestalt formation, the aesthetic or field-resonant perceptions of therapists become more important than diagnostic schemes. Gestalt therapy does not need a normative or evaluative theory of standard human behaviour. Our clients are already able to make contact, albeit in their own (hurting) ways. And they have also been expressing their longing for resonance – in their own ways. The vectors for resonance never disappear because contact is always the first reality of the situation. "It is meaningless to define a breather without air, a walker without gravity and ground" (PHG, 1951/2013, 358), or a situation without contact, or a person without resonance.

The wish, urge, appetite, craving, hunger, desire, passion, lust and striving for a meaningful, resonant exchange with otherness always influence the physical body, the felt body and the wider field. *"All contact is creative adjustment of the organism and environment"* (PHG, 1951/2013, 230), because human beings can never abandon growth completely or irrevocably. The creative possibilities of the therapeutic field offer orientation if we engage in a genuine aesthetic contact with our clients. In a field-centred perspective, contact intentionality and creative adjustment are two core vectors of the field. As gestalt therapists we align ourselves with these forces because they connect us with the field holistically rather than narrowing our perspective to some small allotment. *"Creative adjustment* is in fact the result of this spontaneous strength of survival that allows the individual to be differentiated from the social context, but also to be fully and importantly part of it" (Spagnuolo Lobb, 2013, 44). In field-oriented terms, we can rely on the "self-regulation of a *situational field of contacts"* (ibid., 112).

Our client's need for contact pervades the air because the vectors for resonance have long been part of their field. They also influence other poles, i.e. us. "The abyss in the patient calls to the abyss, the real, unprotected self, in the doctor and not to his confidently functioning security action" (Friedman quoted in Hycner/Jacobs, 1995, 220). Generalising this idea means that our clients' music elicits our own unique melodies. The field's forces, vectors and valences for growth affect us too, as we are another pole of that field. Together we can access them. At the same time, our (physical and phenomenological) resonances are new vectors of the field, posing new affordances. "When our feelings are pronounced invalid, are denied, or go unrecognised by significant others around us, we resort to various ways to manage the double bind of feeling what we should not feel" (Kepner, 2008, 201). This is what our clients have already experienced in one way or another. In therapy they are searching for the resonance of a therapist's whole person, not for a voice at the top end of a couch. These demands on therapists become clearest in the context of *field-centred gestalt therapy*. Since forces for growth have long been vectors of our clients' fields, they can and need to be discovered, tried out, applied, and strengthened in the newly fertilised field created by the encounter. Since gestalt's relational turn, it has become clear that contact is always about shared meaning making: "What many agents of change call resistance is actually, from a forces perspective, a motivational force. Through his 'resistance', the client defends the importance of certain elements of his situation that are overlooked by significant others" (Wollants, 2012, 44). Based on an individualistic paradigm, we see our clients struggling to be seen and recognised. A field-centred perspective informs us about relevant desires for growth which have long been aspects of the situation even if that corner of the field has been ignored and neglected for a considerable time. The analyst and supervisor Oberhoff (2009, 154) thinks that the invitation to "always be on the side of resistance" is phrased much too technically. In more concrete terms, he suggests that "on the part of the supervisee there are not only needs for safety and protection, but also desires for development, which are directed towards reviewing poorly managed relational experiences and coping with them better than before." To me, even this still sounds too much oriented towards deficiencies. I do not see resistances as obstacles or blockades to be bypassed or overcome. They are field markers of unfulfilled resonances pointing at future growth. The field is always fertile.

A clear awareness of growth vectors creates a contagion effect in the therapeutic field, which in turn has an impact on painful and self-restricting views, experiences or behaviour. Roubal (2019, 89) seems to be aware of that when he writes, "Self-support can then appear as a possibility in the shared space of the situation [...] Therefore it would influence the client too. The potentiality of self-support can then open itself also for the client in the situation." In this view, self-support is not a skill taught to clients. It is the aware experience of vectors co-created by therapist and client here, now, and for-next. However, when clients and therapists "realise that this deadness is just one side of the current situation, the aspect which has become a figure, it helps them to focus on those aspects that were in the background until now" (Roubal, 2019, 87 f). On the basis of a consistently field-centred approach, we treat the ground, the rich and fertile field. In other words, the id processes of the situation, i.e. the conditions, affordances, limitations, and opportunities are a foundation for contact and creative growth supporting a co-created 'dance' of therapist and client.

The present field vectors trigger behavioural adjustments and growth. Felt as intentionalities, they aim at expansion, unfolding, development, flourishing and increase, all of which is synonymous with life. This includes an "*expansion* of the habitat", "an increase in *differentiation* of all strata of the habitat", "an increasing *organisation*", and a "change in the general *fluidity* or *rigidity* of the habitat" (Lewin, 1951/2012, 279). It is observable and experienced. In this respect it is the opposite of neurotic regression (ibid., 280 f and 356ff). Contact is the first reality. So growth in field-centred terms can be defined as the unfolding of the field's inherent structural possibilities. This becoming involves the transformation of the field's structure caused by major changes by and to the forces, vectors, and valences. In that sense growth is not a mere metaphor; nor does it refer to some unfolding of an inherent organismic essence. Growth, adaptation, and learning incorporate much more than bringing out a projected authenticity. Germination, sprouting, heightening, thickening, and flowering are necessary for all living beings to survive and flourish. New conditions, limitations or opportunities of the field are experienced as affordances – in therapy, too. Real novelty challenges and creates the (sometimes uncomfortable) urge to change. Often therapy is about what is currently not pleasant or helpful for our clients, what they perceive as burdensome and harmful. But intentions towards resonating contact and growth remain fundamental. At their core, people always aim to "experience new possibilities" (Spagnuolo-Lobb, 2016, 45).

9.3 Self-actualisation in resonance is a key vector of field-centred therapy

For many gestalt therapists, self-regulation is based on the notion of homeostasis: "Thus, the materials and energy of growth are: the conservative attempt of the organism to remain as it has been, the novel environment, the destruction of previous partial equilibria, and the assimilation of something new" (PHG, 1951/2013, 373). In this organismic understanding, the main goal of therapy is the restoration of a self-regulating equilibrium. The image draws on systemic ideas from physics. There "homeostasis is a process of living organisms or organic regulatory systems that essentially consists of keeping physiological quantities constant or within certain permissible limits" (Stangl, 2020). Something similar applies to physical body functions. In both cases, there are processes of adaptation and change that keep the system (e.g. an organism) functional and alive: "*Homeostasis* refers to the coordinated and largely automated physical reactions required to maintain internal states in a living organism" (Damasio, 1999, 39). However, I find it rather questionable whether this is an apt metaphor for human behaviour beyond mere physical survival. Damasio (ibid., 53) suggests, "at their most basic, emotions are part of homeostatic regulation and are poised to avoid the loss of integrity that is a harbinger of death." Many people are forced to endure situations where even their very survival is uncertain. But beyond those fields of destruction, humans aim for more than the avoidance of death and the return to a previous balance. Growth is certainly more than the avoidance of stagnation.

The Portuguese neuroscientist Damasio distinguishes between situations in which an organism deals with pain and those in which it deals with joy. Pleasure "is related to the clever anticipation of what can be done *not* to have a problem. [...] Pleasure, on the other hand, is aligned with reward and is associated with behaviours such as seeking and approaching" (ibid., 78). While a stable equilibrium is certainly the goal of *some* field processes, namely those that ensure survival, most vital processes are not defined by a given zero point which simultaneously functions as the starting and end point of development. In psychological terms: "'Normality' is not what healthy persons aspire to" (Wollants, 2012, 40). Apart from life-threatening situations, human beings are not oriented towards mere life preservation. As *contact* is the first reality, homeostasis is not a 'default setting' of human life and cannot provide a yardstick for successful or happy lives. Goldstein (1934/ 1995, 167 f) stated that there is ultimately only one 'drive': self-actualization. "The organism has definite potentialities, and because it has them it has the need to actualize or realize them. The fulfilment of these needs represents the self-actualization of the organism" (ibid., 239). Since contact is the first reality, the present field vectors create a primal tendency toward actualisation. Fields that are unhampered by inhibiting forces tend towards growth and not just the restitution of a previous balance. "The normal individual is determined by his urge (already inherent in the child) for new experiences, for the conquest of the world, and for an expansion of his sphere of activity in a practical and spiritual sense" (ibid., 238). However, in a *gestalt therapy of the field*, the emphasis is no longer on *self*-realisation of *individual* abilities or on the expression of *inner* abilities. Rather, (human) fields include strong forces for growth through contact and resonance: "We are born, and grow, for and in contact" (Spagnuolo Lobb 2013, 118). And: "Healthy experience is the encounter with the infinite newness of life" (Francesetti et al., 2016, 67). This includes creative adaption at ever higher levels, integration of novelty, and change of the situation in a developmentally open perspective.

Field-centred gestalt therapy is about fostering growth through resonating contact. "Setting the term 'growth' as the goal of therapy springs from the same metaphor as the food analogy. Growth occurs when a body or organism capable of growth assimilates substances from the environment, i.e. nourishes itself" (Blankertz/Doubrawa, 2005, 319). However, self-actualisation presupposes contact with resonating subjects not just with echoing objects. Self-awareness and the development of response-ability cannot take place when resonance is absent or when devaluations, shaming and rejection are prevalent vectors of the field. This is how Spagnuolo Lobb (2018, 432) defines the task of therapy: "Aesthetic Relational Knowledge, in other words, is the *'sensory intelligence' of the shared phenomenological field*. It explains the two spontaneous competences of the therapist at the contact boundary: *embodied empathy and resonance.*" I do not share her distinction between empathy and resonance. Also, I believe a field-centred approach can provide a clearer picture of the tasks. Therapists need to attend to growth vectors already of the situational field. In that sense three points of hers are essential for field-centred therapy:

1 'Sensory intelligence' is but the contagion described above brought about by multiple, field-present, resonant, body-mimetic, micro-processual imitations; it probably also includes resonances with 'atmospheric' constellations, i.e. the affordances or 'ids' of a situation.
2 Both physical and felt bodies are basal: "Only in feeling one's own body is it possible to feel the body of the other and to perceive the potentialities of opening to the other" (Spagnuolo Lobb, 2013, 279).
3 The presence of a therapist changes the client's already fertile field into a new co-created field, rich with potential.

So if a core therapeutic task is to support resonant contact and growth, field-centred gestalt therapists focus on grasping the situation aesthetically, employing their sensory intelligence. Involuntary imitations provide necessary impressions because they are fundamental elements of the shared situation. Unlike an organismic or relational view, *field-centred gestalt therapy* actively utilises awareness of mimicry processes: "The therapist concentrates on the body of the client *and his own body*; he focuses on the sensations he can feel in his own body when he is present with the client" (Wollants, 2012, 82; emphasis by LG). That is rather individualistically phrased. But in my opinion it is not an intervention by one individual (the therapist) affecting the psychic processes of another individual, i.e. the client. Relationally expressed, patients speak about themselves and the therapist, "as the receiver, understands from his own experience in his own special way what he assumes is going on in the patient as the sender. Moreover, the physical expression impresses the receiver and triggers emotional reactions in him" (Geuter, 2015, 273). This contagion, in turn, has an effect on the sender and changes their emotions. This is a rather good representation of the communication process.

Focusing on field resonances not only uncovers and uses possibilities provided by the unfolding field; it also creates new opportunities for growth. Roubal (2019, 85) seems to express this when he writes: A therapist's "experience of freedom, courage and hope now becomes part of the situation, and so the situation itself becomes different." As contact is the first reality of therapy, both client and therapist bring their own vectors (in a manner of speaking). The presence of new poles affect the co-created field right from the start. Hence, therapists do not need to create or push towards something new. Their presence is another vector for discovery, and that is novelty and otherness for the client. Hence, our task as field-centred therapists is to sense the existing structure of the situation, support the forces aiming for growth and explore the joint field with our clients. "Focusing on liveliness already present in the situation brings hope to therapists and helps them cope with their own experience in the presence of a depressed client" (Roubal, 2019, 88). It is crucial to remember that our clients' intentionalities for growth have been present long before therapy began. They provided the impetus for all their creative adaptation processes so far and they have brought these clients to our doorstep. In awareness of the common situation, these vectors now gain new strength and meaning, because aliveness is being in relationships and being in contact with the world. Through resonances of another first-person-singular, clients experience their own vitality. At the same time every living *ex*pression of contact is an *im*pression, too. It is physically perceptible; it evokes contagion reactions, and its reciprocal resonances reinforce precisely those field vectors for growth.

Gestalt therapists in the field take the whole situation into account, with all its conditions, demands, limitations and opportunities. Zinker (1977, 22) described the attitude poetically: "Look at the person the way you would look at a sunset or at mountains. Take in what you see with pleasure. Take in the person for his own sake. After all, you would do that with the sunset too." The whole field – not just the suffering – is a masterpiece, because "it includes both suffering and wishes to overcome it. What makes me vibrate when I look at the client telling me that?" (Spagnuolo Lobb, 2020). That is the core question for any successful therapy. If I concentrate on 'disturbances', I no longer meet my clients as living, resonating subjects. Ultimately I degrade people to symptom carriers and thus to patients in need of my help. They become objects at hand for my therapeutic ambitions. Instead my resonances as a therapist should relate to the sustaining forces of contact and growth because I want to be in contact with novelty, another subject and the whole field. Therapy thus mutates from an occasion for the (healing) revival of pain (cf. Francesetti, 2019, 48) to an occasion for resonant experimentation and experience where it was previously absent and sorely missed.

9.4 In place of a mere therapeutic alliance, resonating contact is the key tool of field-centred therapy

"*Contact, the work that results in assimilation and growth, is the forming of a figure of interest against a ground or context of the organism/environment field*" (PHG, 1951/2013, 231). Since the creation of gestalt therapy, creating a therapeutic alliance has been the bedrock of therapeutic success. According to Schwenkbecher (2019), research has provided ample "evidence that the therapist has a weighty role in the treatment process", and gestalt therapist Robert Resnick (2019, 71) adds that the relationship between the client and the therapist is 30% of the variance of therapy outcome, which research has shown. This is central regardless of modality and it implies that the resonating presence is more important than our acquired professional skills. As such there is more at stake than a 'therapeutic alliance' between two individuals. It affects and effects the whole field and all self-functions. "Personality function operates in two different ways: to support deeper and ever-fuller contact by committing to relationships, values, interests, etc.; or to habitually and defensively avoid unfamiliar contacts by discouraging new awarenesses and relationships" (Philippson, 2009, 21). The question is how to attend to them in therapy.

"The emotional reactions of young children are often influenced by those who are close to them" (Staemmler, 2009, 67). This is no different for adults. A similar process also occurs in therapy, because the *social referencing* that takes place between clients and their therapists "contributes significantly to their becoming themselves" (Dermendzhiyska, 2020, 69). In organismic terms, people process their therapists' contact behaviour including gazes, gestures, posture, etc. (ibid., 78–96). That can be a new and potentially transformative experience. Based on their relational perspective, both Wheeler (2000, 263) and the clinical psychologist Zilcha-Mano (2017, 19) come to the same conclusion: Improvements in the patients' ability to form a satisfactory relationship with the therapist affect their general ability to form better relationships outside of treatment, resulting in a reduction in their presenting symptoms. Perhaps the most succinct expression of the therapeutic importance of resonance phenomena came from Ferenzci: "Without sympathy there is no healing" (in Baer, 2012, 300). Without a subject's own-frequency response, no (re-)structuring of the field can take place. The presence of a therapist changes the mode and quality of contact, although this is not always comfortable or pleasant for either clients or therapists. While some favour supportive, *concordant* contagion as a principal 'tool' of therapy, *complementary* imitation is also helpful as it creates a safe emergency; it fosters a field that includes both supporting and challenging vectors.

Contact always provokes gestalt formation – also in therapy. "It is important for the therapist to support the constitution of the third by acting as a background herself" (Francesetti et al., 2016, 64). What they call a 'third party', I would like to call anchors in the larger field. Again, the fertile field of possibilities comes into view. In Francesetti's field-*oriented* perspective, it is no longer about the *inner* abilities, skills, or knowledge of clients – nor of therapists. For new opportunities of the field to take shape, therapists need to be fully present as persons, not just as professional partners in an alliance. Together with our clients we stabilise, explore and work on the entire fertile field. The starting point is the awareness of sensory contagion processes. In a field-*centred* perspective, therapy is about the flow of unhindered multiple, field-present, resonant, body-mimetic, micro-processual imitations and about the resulting possibilities for a) field exploration, b) the revival of existing vectors, c) the experimentation with new valences, and d) the modification of the fertile field's structure. In this respect, contagion is the resonance of a perceptive pole towards affording field valences. When "Fuchs (2008) estimates that more than a million body signals are exchanged in a therapy session" (Geuter, 2015, 276), this finding points to a significant resource for awareness. Centring our awareness on field processes, therapists are required to respond with their own frequency, i.e. as 'naked' subjects.

Somatic resonance is not a pointer to something. The physical and felt body communicates immediately. As such it provides a direct flow of resonating *im-* and *ex*pressions. In many an individualistic perspective, however, bodywork ultimately only serves an ulterior goal: personal "emotion regulation" (Storch in Storch et al., 2006, 49). However, that perpetuates a Cartesian view focussing the aims of change exclusively on an individual's (inner) abilities. This trimmed understanding supports neoliberal-neoconservative trends towards isolation, alienation, and com- modification. In that view everyone forges their own bodily destiny: "Then the human will gain power over the power centre body" (ibid., 66). Sadly that expresses just more "unrealistic optimism" and "positive illusions" (Kruse, 2017). This as every other self-management approach promotes alienation from one's own body by turning it into an object for augmenta- tion. Although the authors claim that "self-management must not be misunderstood as a call for one's own permanent optimisation" (Storch in Storch et al., 2006, 71), their "Zurich Resource Model" (ibid., 127–142) is but another market offer for self-enhancement that is supposed to create personal 'freedom'. Sadly it taps right into the reduced and uncritical understanding of liberty within liquid modernity. Hence that product enforces the trimming of I-, id-, and personality functions for the purpose of maximising a person's exchange value on liquid markets.

9.5 The use of resonant contagion necessitates a redefinition of countertransference and therapists' training

The field-centred approach affords questions about the education of new gestalt therapists: How can the resonance ability of prospective therapists, and their ability to resonate with field vectors be fostered? Psychoanalytical terminology might provide a clue: Prospective gestalt therapists need to reduce their counter-transference resistance, "which is directed against admitting and taking note of the subjective resonant feelings within oneself" (Oberhoff, 2009, 117). If the sensory perception of 'atmospheric' field constellations is a component of a *gestalt therapy of the field*, the issue of possible counter- transference remains relevant. "We speak of transference when we project introjected basic experiences with significant attachment figures onto current persons in our lives" (Bernstädt/Hahn, 2010, 157). As a special form of projection, this process is part of our basic human make-up. Again in analytical words, "transferences are not pathological reactions in their formal structure, but they are an expression of a natural human tendency that serves survival" (Oberhoff, 2009, 57). If people were not able to transfer their own experiences to new situations, they could not adapt or grow. Transference becomes problematic however when past (traumatic) experiences – i.e. limiting and inhibiting field vectors – hinder awareness about the conditions, demands, limitations and opportunities of a current situation.

Francesetti et al. (2016, 74) state that previously unacquired skills emerge in therapy as a need for a specific and new contact experience. "This is the relational need that the patient wants to satisfy or become aware of and acknowledge in therapy. This is her disturbed contact intentionality and at the same time it is her story and her next step." In other words, expanding the perception of field vectors should be a key orientation point of therapy and the training of new therapists. Gestalt therapists need to focus their awareness on liminal processes, improving their negative capability, more than they have to date. By the same token, it behooves us to be as clear as possible about our own needs and feelings so that these do not leak unknowingly into the therapeutic process. That means our own intentions, etc., can cloud clear sensory awareness of the forces, vectors and valences relevant for our clients' growth. In this context Bernstädt and Hahn (2010, 161 f) make a very helpful distinction between 'transference shadows' and 'projective perceptions'. For them, the former constitutes an attempt to introduce a therapist's own issues into the therapeutic situation while the latter is a "a way of accessing the reality" of the client and the field. Similarly, the body therapist Geuter (2015, 305–307) distinguishes between "personal countertransference" on the one hand in which one's own psychic material is focused and an "induced countertransference" or "counterfeeling" on the other hand. Overall, I find the terms transference and countertransference quite unhelpful for the description of field processes because they are based on individualistic paradigms. When it comes to the perception of multiple, field-present, resonant, body-mimetic, micro-processual imitations, I rather speak of contagion. In any case, this involves the joint 'digestion' of resonances and a co-created meaning making. The prerequisite for this is that the therapist "concentrates on the contact with his counterpart with all his senses and at the same time perceives his own resonance with relaxed attention" (Bernstädt/Hahn, 2010, 161). All vectors are potentially relevant. When a therapist's reactions have nothing to do with the experience and life of a client as present in the therapeutic situation they limit awareness. Hence only certain aspects of the field become figure. Unfortunately, it is not immediately obvious at first whether a therapist's resonance is helping or hindering. In order to foster the therapeutic process of separating the sheep from the goats through negotiation and meaning-making the training of prospective therapists needs to focus much more on their skills to use liminal perceptions.

At the same time, sceptics note, "We experience an almost euphoric revaluation of countertransference, as an extremely important perceptual instrument" (Oberhoff, 2009, 114). I think this is valid if we do not differentiate clearly between resonance processes and countertransference: "Countertransference is a state in which I experience without knowing" (Bollas, 1987, quoted in ibid., 187). Here the British psychoanalyst describes the *unaware* experience of a common field, but confusingly calls this countertransference. Being liminal processes par excellence, both resonance and countertransference are phenomena at first that we are unaware of. Yet the ability to perceive physical and emotional contagion and to make them aware, is fundamental for the growth of the field and for the success of therapy. It is vital for both client and therapist to become more fully aware of their common situation and explore new possibilities of gestalt formation and field modulation. The resonance behaviour of a field-centred therapist is a decisive element of this process. However, since a clear mental or emotional sorting of impressions is hardly possible at first, therapists have a special responsibility not to impose their own themes and views on their clients. And yet, a fractional, controlled, or selective resonance with only a part of the multiple, field-present, resonant, body-mimetic, micro-processual imitations is impossible. Since we can hardly suppress or stop the physical manifestations of our resonances, they are part of the field long before we become aware of them. We cannot simply bracket our contagion reactions until the next session with our supervisor. Of course, we can refuse to become aware of situational resonances. In doing so however we restrict the conditions, demands, limitations and opportunities of the therapeutic situation – and we risk the client's transference and at worst a repetition of old traumatising experiences. Here is one question that needs further study, I believe: How can we distinguish counter-transferences from resonances while being fully present and focusing on the resonating field?

9.6 Conclusion

For a *gestalt therapy of the field*, "*resonance desire*" (Rosa, 2019a, 195) is of central importance. An aesthetic attitude, sensory intelligence, etc., describe a therapeutic approach that focuses on field resonances. Seen from an individualistic paradigm perspective, however, the multiple, field-present, resonant, body-mimetic, micro-processual imitations would merely be another set of diagnostic tools. Instead, they are an inevitably human mode of response to a meaningful counterpart. Resonance is always an essential intentionality of the field because humans are subjects, not objects 'to hand'. They need genuine reactions from other first-person-singulars to 'come to themselves'. The intentionality to resonate and the desire to be resonated is part of the humane condition because contact is the first reality. "Conversely, a lack of resonance or desynchronisation of brain rhythms corresponds to insufficient environmental coherence: if the human being cannot resonate with the world, it remains closed to him, mute, and he remains incomprehensible to himself, alien" (Scheurle, 2017, 45). The vectors towards contact, novelty and growth can be overwritten by experiences where resonance is either lacking or shamed, belittled and negated. I agree with Jacobs when she states, "I believe that underlying many, perhaps all self-object functions, is a deep yearning for genuine encounter with others. As therapists we may begin with self-object functions, but not *end* there" (Hycner/Jacobs, 1995, 205).

Since contact is the first reality, resonances are fundamental vectors and valences; subjects are the perceptive poles of fields. This relates to body processes that are scientifically verifiable as much as to the felt body we explore phenomenologically. Human beings are always *of* the field. Therefore, all their experiences, knowledge, abilities, skills, and resources are present even when they cannot be part of the gestalt formation. With awareness based on support, new figures emerge and the ground can (re-) gain stability. Based on that view, the burden is no longer on the individual to close their personal old gestalts through re-experiencing or relating in some mystical 'in-between'. Healing processes *of* the field and growth become possible when relevant forces and valences are supported. Thus for (gestalt) therapy it is vital that we improve our ability to focus in the field, remain in a liminal state and be (rather than act) in the presence of our clients.

Note

1   *PHG, 1951/2013, 421.*

Chapter 10

Epilogue

The field-centred gestalt approach is necessarily based on considerations of the social embeddedness of therapy. "The 11th commandment is: Thou shalt not be indifferent", said Marian Turski, survivor of the Shoah, in his speech at the memorial service in Auschwitz-Birkenau on 27th January 2020 (in Freedland, 2020). Resonance, this human quest for an active response of others, is fundamental for me personally, for gestalt therapy, and for a society where people will no longer see each other as commodities. Regardless of whether one interprets today's society as postmodern, late capitalist, free-market, neoliberal, neoconservative, or liquid, the advancing alienation, increasing structural weakness of peoples' fields, and a desensitisation towards affective resonances, are noticeable consequences. In liquid modernity, normality remains an elusive commodity. Moreover, the market mechanisms that pervade all aspects of life have created more and more instabilities. They are being analysed and felt. It seems societal realities as well as I-, id-, and personality functions have accelerated into a "permacrisis" (Zuleeg et al., 2021).

10.1 The COVID-19 pandemic

Especially – but not exclusively – those working in nursing and medical professions caught very intense "glimpses of the immense human cost of the pandemic, the great well of loss, fear, sadness and grief beneath the mounting statistics" (O'Hagan, 2020). Even before the COVID-19 pandemic, studies showed that working in intensive care increased the likelihood of developing post-traumatic stress disorder by 20% (ibid.). Traumatisation has become a structurally embedded vector of the current societal situation. The prolonged stay in traumatic fields affects all poles of that field. Due to the prevalent ideology, however, it is experienced as something inside individuals. Starting from a field-centred perspective, it is not surprising that the experience of COVID-19 has "elevated rates of stress or anxiety, [...] loneliness, depression, harmful alcohol and drug use, and self-harm or suicidal behaviour are expected to rise" (ibid.). The consequences will be felt long after contact bans

DOI: 10.4324/9781003454809-11

have been lifted, not least because rich and poor nations as well as rich and poor people within different societies are affected unequally (cf. Cassidy, 2020). These inducers of psychological stress come on top of those typical for the liquid modern era. When stress-management is being individualised it is no wonder that violent behaviour has increased: "According to a special report by the British government, at least 16 women and children have been killed at home in the three weeks since the curfew began on 23 March. Normally it would have been 'only' five women" (Schulz, 2020; see also Betschka, 2020; Fetscher, 2020; and Althammer, 2020). As therapists and fellow human beings: How are we going to respond?

10.2 Planetary destruction

"Now an increasing number of psychologists believe the trauma that is a consequence of climate breakdown is also one of the biggest obstacles in the struggle to take action against rising greenhouse gas emissions." (Ambrose, 2020). The menace of global extinction produces widespread trauma, not only among younger people. There is a growing sense that this needs (also) a therapeutic response for people to move beyond paralysis. As human-made global destruction looms, it evades the control of individuals, single societies, and even transnational organisations. Living with ungovernable threats triggers fear; it dramatically reduces a person's sense of agency and induces resonance fatigue. "According to a study the richest one percent of the world's population produce more than twice as many climate-damaging carbon dioxide emissions as the poorer half of humanity combined." (Zeit online, 2020). This article referred to a report published by the development organisation Oxfam ahead of the general debate of the 75th UN General Assembly in New York. That may be another reason why solutions are easy to describe and so very hard to implement politically. Ever since modernity began, the commodity frontier has been moved on and on, trashing the planet and hiding the money. That isn't an aberration – it is capitalism (Monbiot, 2021).

10.3 Another war – now in Europe

War is recurring as a means of politics – in Europe, too. While that is devastating for many people in Ukraine, it is not as surprising as commenta-tors make out. Modernity never reduced the number of wars while it expanded the technical possibilities and thus the viciousness of wars. Killing and its accompanying atrocities had previously been relocated to the so-called theatres of war, i.e. to other (non-white) parts of the globe. Yes, European solidarity with the Ukrainian victims of war and war crimes has been exceptional. Unfortunately, there is a whiff of racism about it, which has been noticed by those living in the 'usual' war zones (Gathara, 2022).

Disconcertingly antisemitic and racist tendencies have been penetrating the mainstream of the body politic in several liquid modern societies, while the same societies have largely been in denial about their own structural racism (Bouie, 2022). What really makes the war in Ukraine a new phenomenon is the fact that nuclear powers are in (almost) direct confrontation with each other. Instead of ubiquitous proxy wars, the possibility of nuclear annihilation is back as a figure forming from that ground.

10.4 The internal 'crisis of democracy'

Cui bono? Who benefits from these developments – apart from dictators, self-enriching oligarchs, and right-wing populists? Robert Reich, former Secretary of Labour in the Clinton administration calculated that Jeff Bezos could give $105,000 to each Amazon employee and still be as rich as he was before the Covid-19 pandemic (Neate, 2020a). Quite a few Western capitalists have not only been less affected by the pandemic; they have increased their profit margins (see Collins et al., 2020; also Neate, 2020b). The extra wealth of the world's richest (white) men amounts to more than what the British government is estimated to have spent on tackling the pandemic and the subsequent economic damage that has been wrought on the country's 66 million people (Editorial, *The Guardian*, 2020). During the same period, more than 200,000 Americans have died and over 50 million people have lost their jobs in the so-called richest country on earth. As therapists and fellow human beings: How are we going to respond?

"Misinformation and dangerous conspiracy theories thrive when people are stressed and alone" (Taylor, 2020). Facts are doubted because they contradict personal feelings and preconceived beliefs. In his novel *1984* George Orwell wrote: "Reality is not external. Reality exists in the human mind, and nowhere else. [...] Whatever the party holds to be truth, is truth" (quoted in d'Ancona, 2017). This is liquid-individualistic constructivism with a vengeance. If I see the sun rising on the horizon every morning, the earth must be flat ... For individuals it becomes increasingly hard to distinguish real from so-called alternative facts and knowledgeable experts from opinionated individuals or state-funded trolls. The "liquefaction of fact-based reporting" (Taylor, 2020) is being driven by those who

- benefit from liquid normality, like corporate business enterprises;
- intend to undermine or limit 'woke' democracy to build their own empire, like for example governments in Russia, Hungary, China, Brazil, India, Britain, the USA;
- profit from the insecurity of many people, such as right-wing ideologues, white supremacists, and Nazis.

Disinformation, irrationality, and mysticism are by no means inventions of today's anti-modernists. In the wake of the European plagues after 1348, the ardent search for scapegoats often took the form of racism and anti-Semitic pogroms. But wherever objective, observable, repeatable methods of verification are demonised or criminalised, *post*modernity bears striking similarities to the *pre*modern Dark Ages. When subjective opinions or unverified government propaganda are seen as having the same value as empirical science, facts become just another construct or a grand old narrative.

On the other hand, death and destruction on a global scale whether by pandemic, war or environmental extinction might bring back evidence-based governing as an effective way to respond to real threats. The current 'riders of the apocalypse' expose the fact that the threat of extinction is not an individual construct but a social product. The permacrisis is exposing the limitations of liquid-modern markets and the inadequacy of neoliberal or neoconservative ideologies. Markets are failing not because of scams like insider trading or corporate fraud. "A failure occurs when the marketplace allocates resources in a way that does not optimally deliver wellbeing" (Devine, 2020). When it comes to the global destruction of the environment, the so-called 'free' market is unable to regulate because, contrary to neo-conservative beliefs, market forces are "neither neutral nor universal. They partly mirror a society's evolving norms and values. But they also reflect who in society has the most power to make or influence the underlying market rules" (Reich, 2020). Neither liberté, égalité, and fraternité nor even the survival of our species is manufactured by market transactions alone. They depend on community-related resonances for liberty, equality, justice, and change.

Moving beyond liquid modernity, we need to redefine our understanding of freedom. The German philosopher Redecker (2020) wrote,

"One apparently only feels one's freedom when one can use it savagely: Freedom of expression can only be felt by being allowed to hurt others, freedom of consumption by being able to drive in petrol guzzlers, and freedom of public movement by being allowed to cough in other people's faces. The liberal freedom of choice is already a rather narrow horizon of freedom, but here it becomes even more authoritarian. [...] In my eyes, this attitude is based on the fact that we have conceived the modern citizen according to the model of the owner who can do as he pleases in his own domain."

Hyper-individualistic freedom means to assert and live out one's own interests in competition with and at the expense of others. This narcissistic art of the deal is the opposite of resonance and responsibility.

Still, the future is not clear, because "as soon as there is a power relation, there are possibilities of contradiction. We are never completely trapped by power; under certain conditions and with a precise strategy, one can always avert its grip" (Foucault quoted in Grubner, 2017, 121). Perhaps modernity is not over after all. It certainly awaits its remodelling. Conceivably we can reform our obsession with material growth and consumerism as we become aware of the real price: alienation, threats of (nuclear) war, possibly more global pandemics, and impending planetary collapse. What could or should this mean for gestalt therapy?

"Consequently, what is widespread today is a fear of death (from an early age) and a need for rootedness. The clinical outcome that we see in our clients is a sort of anaesthesia" (Spagnuolo Lobb, 2017, 50). The permacrisis has exaggerated that trend towards desensitisation, narcissism and dissociative states supported by the habit of staying with our smartphones, and an inability to meet our neighbours or to help our children to make sense of their lives. It is precisely the ubiquitous alienation from others that engenders insecurity and fear, that leads to pathological reactions individually, and to political irrationalities socially. Therapy is certainly not a resistance movement. Yet, what happens in therapy rooms doesn't stay in therapy rooms. Strengthening awareness has an effect beyond our doors.

Do gestalt therapists "work largely to ensure that individuals become (or remain) what they are supposed to be in the sense of neoliberal conceptions of the subject, namely free, cost-benefit calculating entrepreneurs of themselves" (Grubner, 2017, 251)? Or do we strengthen the human capacity to respond, i.e. our own and our clients' "response-ability" (Perls in Binderman, 1974, 287)? Situations of complex danger afford traumatic reactions. In order to stabilise the ground and avoid such traumas, therapy should aim to promote

1   measurable safety,
2   felt reassurance,
3   experienced self-efficacy and resonant collective effectuality,
4   contact, connection and resonance, as well as
5   hope (cf. Behring/Eichenberg, 2020, 23).

Here, now and regarding next steps, I believe gestalt therapy can contribute to a new balance between autonomy and community, as any humanist therapy should. Adopting a field-centred paradigm feels like a necessary next step. We, the practitioners of gestalt therapy should be the first to foster creative experimentation. We should use our own sense of daring, of being unabashedly bold. We need to grow in order to be agents for change in liquid modern times. And we need to focus on the broader field in order to be response-able.

Literature

ADORNO, THEODOR W. / FRENKEL-BRUNSWIK, ELSE / LEVINSON, DANIEL J. / SANFORD, R. NEVITT (1950): *The Authoritarian Personality*. Harper und Brothers, New York.

AKOUN, D. / HEINZMANN, R. (2021): Gestalttherapie und Politik – Ein kurzer Einblick in Theorie und Praxis, *Geschichte und Gegenwart*, downloaded on 30 March 2021 from www.dvg-gestalt.de/wp-content/uploads/2021/03/2-Politik-und-gestalttherapie-09-25_2.pdf.

ALLOA, E. / DEPRAZ, N. (2012): Edmund Husserl – "Ein merkwürdig unvollkommen konstituiertes Ding", in Alloa, E. / Bedorf, T. / Grüny, C. / Klass, T.N. (eds.): *Leiblichkeit*, 7–22.

ALTHAMMER, R. (2020): Corona-Krise in Berlin: Deutlich mehr Einsätze wegen häuslicher Gewalt, *aber kaum mehr Anzeigen*, rbb24, 21 April 2020 downloaded on 14 June 2020 from www.rbb24.de.

AMBROSE, J. (2020): 'Hijacked by anxiety': How climate dread is hindering climate action, The Guardian, 8 October 2020, downloaded on 6 November 2020 from www.theguardian.com.

AMENDT-LYON, N. (2018): The Boundaries of Gestalt Therapy and the Limits of Our Imagination: Hermann Schmitz's Adolf Hitler in History and "New Phenomenology", *Gestalt Review*, Vol. 22, No. 3, 302–330.

AMENDT-LYON, N. (2019): The world-bearing naught, in Perls, F. / Robine, J.M. / Bowman, C. (eds.): *Psychopathology of Awareness*, 171–177.

APPEL-OPPER, J. (2010): Relational Living Body Psychotherapy: From Physical Resonances to Embodied Interventions and Experiments, *The USA Body Psychotherapy Journal*, Vol. 1, No. 1, 51–56.

APPEL-OPPER, J. (2011): Relationale Körper-zu-Körper-Kommunikation in der Psychotherapie, *Zeitschrift Psychoanalyse und Körper*, Vol. 18, 10.Jg., No. 1, 65–71.

APPEL-OPPER, J. (2017): Heilsame Körperdialoge im interkörperlichen Feld – Interventionen und Experimente, *Gestalttherapie*, Vol. 31, No. 2, 55–74.

APPEL-OPPER, J. (2018): Everybody has his/her own melody. Dialogue with Nora Astrup Dahm, *Gestaltterapeut Forenning*, 1/2018, downloaded on 2 November 2019 from www.ngfo.no.

ATKIN, E. (2018): Do you know where your healing crystals come from?, *The New Republic*, 11 May 2018, downloaded on 29 April 2021 from https://newrepublic.com/article/148190/know-healing-crystals-come-from.

AWAD, A. (2021): The new age looks enlightened and exotic because it borrows freely from non-Anglo cultures, *The Guardian*, 25 April 2021, downloaded on 29 April 2021 from www.theguardian.com.

BAER, U. (2012): *Kreative Leibtherapie.* Das Lehrbuch.

BAKEWELL, S. (2016): Think big, be free, have sex … 10 reasons to be an existentialist, *The Guardian*, 4 March 2016, downloaded on 16 April 2020 from www.theguardian.com.

BARRETT-IBARRIA, S. (2020): Cam girl reality: An enticing illusion leaves many models poor and defeated, *The Guardian*, 14 January 2020, downloaded on 14 January 2020 from www.theguardian.com.

BAUMANN, Z. (2000): Liquid Modernity.

BAUMANN, Z. (2011): No one is in control. That is the major source of contemporary fear, 6 September 2011, www.youtube.com/watch?v=73Nmv-4jvSc.

BAUMANN, Z. (2012): Flüchtige Zeiten: Leben in der Ungewissheit, Alles in (Un-)Ordnung? Neue Unübersichtlichkeiten in einer globalisierten Welt, 16. Karlsruher Gespräche, Symposium 11 February 2012, www.youtube.com/watch?v=YyyvCdR9MPg

BBC BOOKS. (1996): *The Nation's Favourite Poems.*

BECKER, R. (2019): Das ängstliche Selbst oder der kurze weg vom Ideal der Selbstverwirklichung zum Zwang der Autonomie, *Gestalttherapie*, 2/2019, 29–41.

BEHRING, R. / EICHENBERG, C. (eds.). (2020): Die Psyche in Zeiten der Corona-Krise, *Herausforderungen und Lösungsansätze für Psychotherapeuten und soziale Helfer.*

BEISSER, A. (1970): The Paradoxical Theory of Change, in Fagan, J. / Sheperd, I. (eds.): *Gestalt Therapy Now.*

BERNSTÄDT, J. (2017): Über den Umgang mit Scham und Widerstand in der Gestalttherapie – eine Einführung, *Gestalttherapie*, 2/2017, 11–19.

BERNSTÄDT, J. / HAHN, S. (2010): *Gestalttherapie mit Gruppen.*

BETSCHKA, J. (2020): Coronavirus-Maßnahmen in Berlin Kriminalität sinkt insgesamt, aber häusliche Gewalt nimmt zu, Der Tagesspiegel, 26 March 2020, downloaded on 14 June 2020 from www.tagesspiegel.de.

BINDERMAN, R.M. (1974): The Issue of Responsibility in Gestalt Therapy, *Psychotherapy: Theory, Research and Practice*, Vol. 11, No. 3, Fall 1974, 287–288.

BISCHOF-KÖHLER, D. (1989): *Spiegelbild und Empathie.*

BLANKERTZ, S. (2012): Gestalttherapie. Essentials. Das wichtigste aus dem Grundlagenwerk von Perls, Goodman, Hefferline.

BLANKERTZ, S. / DOUBRAWA, E. (2005): *Lexikon der Gestalttherapie.*

BOCIAN, B. (2010): Fritz Perls in Berlin 1893–1933: Expressionism – Psychoanalysis – Judaism.

BOCIAN, B. (2019): From character analysis to interpersonal psychoanalysis to gestalt therapy, in Perls, F. / Robine, J.M. / Bowman, C. (eds.): *Psychopathology of Awareness*, 105–136.

BOECKH, A. (2019): Die dialogische Struktur des Selbst, *Perspektiven einer relationalen und emotionsorientierten Gestalttherapie.*

BOGHOSSIAN, P. (2006): Fear of Knowledge. Against Relativism and Constructivism.

BOLLAS, C. (1987): Der Schatten des Objekts. Das ungedachte Bekannte: Zur Psychoanalyse der frühen Entwicklung.

BOOTH, R. (2020): Data on Covid care home deaths kept secret 'to protect commercial interests', *The Guardian*, 27 August 2020, downloaded on 20 August 2020 from www.theguardian.com.

BOUIE, J. (2022): The Backlash against C.R.T. shows that Republicans are losing ground, *New York Times*, 4 February 2022, downloaded on 26 March 2022 from www.nytimes.com.

BOURDIEU, P. (1982): Die feinen Unterschiede.

BOURDIEU, P. (1997): Der Tote packt den Lebenden.

BOWMAN, C. (2019): A missing link in the evolution of gestalt therapy, in Perls, F. / Robine, J.-M. / Bowman, C. (eds.): *Psychopathology of Awareness*, 57–64.

BRANDMEYER, K. / PIRCK, P. / POGODA, A. / ALTHANNS, L. (2011): Markenkraft zum Nulltarif: Der Trick mit den Resonanzfeldern.

BREITHAUPT, F. (2009): Kulturen und Empathie.

BRIELER, U. (2005): Der neoliberale Charakter, *Freitag*, 2 December 2005, downloaded on 30 August 2020 von www.freitag.de/autoren/der-freitag/der-neoliberale-charakter.

BREUER, H. (2002): Zellen die Gedanken lesen, in Geist & Gehirn, *Spektrum der Wissenschaft*, 02/2002.

BUBER, M. (1922/1979): Ich und Du.

CAIN, S. (2011): Still – Die Bedeutung von Introvertierten in einer lauten Welt.

CASSIDY, A. (2020): Rassismus und Corona: Tödliche Ungleichheit, *Süddeutsche Zeitung*, 10 April 2020, downloaded on 14 June 2020 from www.sueddeutsche.de.

CLAID, E. (2018): Between You and Me, in Spagnuolo Lobb, M., et al. (eds.): *The Aesthetic of Otherness: Meeting at the Boundary in a Desensitized World*. Proceedings, 161–170.

COLE, P. (2019): Fritz Perls: wounded visionary of the perennial philosophy, in Perls, F. / Robine, J.M. / Bowman, C. (eds.): *Psychopathology of Awareness*, 157–169.

COCOZZA, P. (2018): No hugging: Are we living through a crisis of touch?, *The Guardian*, 7 May 2018, downloaded on 16 April 2020 from www.theguardian.com.

COLLINS, C. / OCAMPO, O. / PASLASKI, S. (2020): Billionaire Bonanza, Wealth Windfalls, Tumbling Taxes, and Pandemic Profiteers, *Institute for Policy Studies*, 23 April 2020.

CRAMER, F. (1996): *Symphonie des Lebendigen*. Versuch einer allgemeinen Resonanztheorie.

DAMASIO, A. (1999): *The Feeling of What Happens*. Body and Emotion in the Making of Consciousness.

D'ANCONA, M. (2017): Ten alternative facts for the post truth world, *The Guardian*, 12 May 2017, downloaded on 15 September 2020 from www.theguardian.com.

DERMENDZHIYSKA, E. (2020): How you attach to people may explain a lot about your inner life, *The Guardian*, 10 January 2020, downloaded on 14 January 2020 from www.theguardian.com.

DESMOND, B. (2018): Soma-aesthetic group therapy: Moving bodies, changing lives, in Spagnuolo Lobb, M., et al. (eds.): *The Aesthetic of Otherness: Meeting at the Boundary in a Desensitized World*. Proceedings, 181–192.

DEVINE, R.S. (2020): The 'market' won't save us from climate disaster. We must rethink our system, *The Guardian*, 19 November 2020, downloaded on 20 November 2020 from www.theguardian.com.

DGPPN (Deutsche Gesellschaft für Psychiatrie und Psychotherapie, Psychosomatik und Nervenheilkunde). (2019): Zahlen und Fakten der Psychiatrie und Psychotherapie, downloaded on 19 January 2020 von www.dgppn.de/schwerpunkte/zahlenundfakten.html.

DIEZ, T. (2006): Postmoderne Ansätze, in Schieder, S. / Spindler, M. (eds.): *Theorien der Internationalen Beziehungen*, 473ff.

DREITZEL, P. (2004): Gestalt und Prozess. Eine psychotherapeutische Diagnostik oder: Der gesunde Mensch hat wenig Charakter, *Reflexive Sinnlichkeit II*.

DREITZEL, P. (2007): Emotionale Gewahrsein. Die mensch-Umwelt-Beziehung aus gestalttherapeutischer Sicht, *Reflexive Sinnlichkeit I*.

EAGLETON, T. (1996): The Illusions of Postmodernism.

EDITORIAL. (2020): The Guardian view on shameless CEOs: because they're worth it? 18 December 2020, downloaded on 18 December 2020 from www.theguardian.com.

EHRENBERG, A. (2004): Das erschöpfte Selbst: Depression und Gesellschaft in der Gegenwart.

ELIAS, N. (1980): Über den Prozess der Zivilisation (2 volumns).

FARRELLY, F. (1974): *Provocative Therapy*. Shields Publishing Company.

FERRARIS, M. (2014): *Manifest des Neuen Realismus*.

FETSCHER, C. (2020): Corona und die Ausgehbeschränkungen: Häusliche Gewalt ist kein Schicksal - sondern ein Problem, *das alle angeht*, Zeit online, 12 April 2020, downloaded on 14 June 2020 from www.zeit.de.

FRANCESETTI, G. (ed.). (2015): *Absence Is the Bridge between Us*.

FRANCESETTI, G. (2019): A clinical exploration of atmospheres: Towards a field-based clinical practice, in Francesetti, G. / Griffero, T. (eds.): *Psychopathology and Atmospheres: Neither Inside Nor Outside*, 35–68.

FRANCESETTI, G. (2020): Die Feldperspektive in der klinischen Praxis, *Gestalttherapie*, 1/2020, 41–66.

FRANCESETTI, G. / GRIFFERO, T. (eds.). (2019): *Psychopathology and Atmospheres: Neither Inside Nor Outside*.

FRANCESETTI, G. / GECELE, M. / ROUBAL, J. (2016): Psychopathologie: Ein gestalttherapeutischer Ansatz, in Francesetti, G. / Gecele, M. / Roubal, J. (eds.): *Gestalttherapie in der klinischen Praxis*. Von der Psychopathologie zur Ästhetik des Kontakts, 59–75.

FRANCESETTI, G. / KERRY-REED, E. / VÁZQUEZ-BANDIN, C. (2019): Obsessive-Compulsive Experiences: A Gestalt Therapy Perspective.

FRAMBACH, L. (1996): Salomo Friedländer / Mynona (1871–1946). Ausgrabung einer fast vergessenen Quelle der Gestalttherapie, *Gestalttherapie*, 1/1996, 3–23.

FREEDLAND, J. (2020): 'Thou shalt not be indifferent': From Auschwitz's gate of hell, a last, desperate warning, *The Guardian*, 27 January 2020, downloaded on 27 January 2020 from www.theguardian.com.

FRIEDLÄNDER, S. (2009): Schöpferische Indifferenz (1918, 1926), in Geerken, H. / Thiel, D. (eds.): *Gesammelte Schriften Band 10*.

FROMM, E. (1977): Gespräch mit Micaela Lämmle und Jürgen Lodemann, *Erich Fromm Study Center Berlin – EFSC*, www.youtube.com/watch?v=L_2mn39AU0c, 6 May 2021.

FROMM, E. / SUZUKI, D.T. / DE MARTINO, R. (1972): Zen-Buddhismus und Psychoanalyse.

FUCHS, T. (2000a): Leib-Raum-Person. Entwurf einer Phänomenologischen Anthropologie.

FUCHS, T. (2000b): *Psychopathologie von Leib und Raum*. Phänomenologisch-empirische Untersuchung zu depressiven und paranoiden Erkrankungen.

FUCHS, T. (2008): Phänomenologische Spurensuche in der psychiatrischen Diagnostik, in Wollschläger, M. (ed.): *Hirn – Herz – Seele – Schmerz*. Psychotherapie zwischen Neurowissenschaften und Geisteswissenschaften, 55–68.

FUCHS, T. (2019a): The uncanny as atmosphere, in Francesetti, G. / Griffero, T. (eds.): *Psychopathology and Atmospheres: Neither Inside Nor Outside*, 101–118.

FUCHS, T. (2019b): Phänomenales Feld und Lebensraum. Skizze einer phänomenalen Konzeption der Psychotherapie, *Gestalttherapie*, 2/2019, 114–129.

FUHR, R. / SRECKOVIC, M. / GREMMLER-FUHR, M. (2001): Handbuch der Gestalttherapie.

GALIMBERTI, U. (1989): Il corpo.

GALTUNG, J. (1969): Violence, Peace, and Peace Research, *Journal of Peace Research*, Vol. 6, No. 3, 167–191.

GATHARA, P. (2022): Covering Ukraine: A mean streak of racist exceptionalism, *Al Jazeera*, 1 March 2022, downloaded on 26 March 2022 from www.aljazeera.com/opinions/2022.

GECELE, M. (2019): Chasing joy in the liquid time of emptiness: Obsessive compulsive experiences in postmodern era, in Francesetti et al. (ed.): *Obsessive-Compulsive Experiences: A Gestalt Therapy Perspective*, 313–327.

GEUTER, U. (2015): *Körperpsychotherapie*. Grundriss einer Theorie für die klinische Praxis.

GIBSON, J.J. (1979): The Ecological Approach to Visual Perception.

GINDL, B. (2002): Die Resonanz der Seele.

GOLDSTEIN, K. (1934/1995): The Organism.

GRAMSCI, A. (1930): Prison Notebooks.

GRAY, J. (2017): Post truth by Matthew D'Ancona and Post-Truth by Evan Davis review – Is this really a new era of politics?, *The Guardian*, 19 May 2017, downloaded on 16 September 2020 from www.theguardian.com.

GRUBNER, A. (2017): Die Macht der Psychotherapie im Neoliberalismus: Eine Streitschrift.n

GUTJAHR, L. (2016): Corporal concernedness or contact? Gestalt Therapy and the 'New Phenomenology', *Gestalt Journal of Australia and New Zealand*, November 2016, 19–42.

GUTJAHR, L. (2018): Nourishing Notions or Poisonous Propositions? Can "New Phenomenology" Inspire Gestalt Therapy?, *Gestalt Review*, Vol. 22, No. 3, 331–357.

HABERMAS, J. (1980): Die Moderne – ein unvollendetes Projekt, *Die Zeit*, No. 39/1980, downloaded on 29 March 2020 from www.zeit.de.

HATFIELD, E. / CACIOPPO, J.T. / RAPSON, R.L. (1994): Emotional Contagion.

HAY, D.F. (1994): Prosocial development, *Journal of Child Psychology and Psychiatry and Allied Disciplines*, Vol. 35, 29–71.

HEBRON, S. (2014): John Keats and 'negative capability', 15 May 2014, downloaded on 7 January 2020 from www.bl.uk.

HENNING, C. (2015): *Theorien der Entfremdung*. Zur Einführung.

HOFFMAN, M.L. (2000): Empathy and moral development: Implications for caring and justice.

HOGREBE, W. (2006): Echo des Nichtwissens.

HUME, D. (1739): A Treatise on Human Nature, Book I, Of the Understanding, Part I, Section I, accessed on 30 March 2022 on https://davidhume.org/texts/t/1/1/1.

HUSSERL, E. (1987): Essays and Lectures 1911–1921, *Husserliana XXV*.

HYCNER, R. / JACOBS, L. (1995): The Healing Relationship in Gestalt Therapy, *A Dialogic / Self Psychology Approach*.

INGOLD, T. (1993): The temporality of the landscape, *World Archaeology*, Vol. 25, No. 2, 153–174, downloaded on 10 February 2020 from www.tandfonline.com/doi/abs/10.1080/00438243.1993.9980235.

JACOBS, L. (2017): Hopes, Fears and Enduring Relational Themes, *British Gestalt Journal*, Vol. 26, No. 1, 7–16.

JAEGGI, R. (2016): *Entfremdung*. Zur Aktualität eines sozialphilosophischen Problems.

JULMI, C. / RAPPE, G. (2018): Atmosphärische Führung. Stimmungen wahrnehmen und gezielt beeinflussen.

JURKSTAITE-PACEESIENE, L. / SORAKA, A. / MILIKAUSKIENE, D. / KRETSCHMER, K. / SAPEZINSKIENE, L. (2018): The experience of relationship in the Argentine Tango: 'Haptics' concepts and gestalt experience cycle, in Spagnuolo Lobb, M., et al. (eds.): *The Aesthetic of Otherness: Meeting at the Boundary in a Desensitized World*. Proceedings, 265–278.

JUNG, M. (2001): *Hermeneutik*. Zur Einführung.

KAISER, G. (2016): Auf dem Weg in die Knechtschaft, Buchbesprechung zu Rosa, H. (2016): Resonanz. Eine Soziologie der Weltbeziehung, 21 November 2016, downloaded on 19 January 2020 from www.literaturkritik.de.

KENNEDY, D. (2003): The Phenomenal World, *The British Gestalt Journal*, Vol. 12, No. 2, 76–87.

KEPNER, J. (2008): Body Process.

KEPNER, J. (2016): The Relational Nervous System in gestalt Body Process Psychotherapy, Presentation at AAGT/EAGT Conference in Taormina, downloaded on 1 November 2019 von www.jimkepner.com.

KOHUT, H. (1981a): Die Heilung des Selbst.

KOHUT, H. (1981b): Reflections on Empathy, downloaded on 18 April 2021 from www.youtube.com/watch?v=ZQ6Y3hoKI8U.

KRUSE, M. (2017): The power of Trump's positive thinking, The president always has believed he could will himself to success. But has he crossed the line between optimism and delusion? Politico Magazine, 13 October 2017, downloaded on 6 December 2020 from www.politico.com.

KUHN, T. (1973): Die Struktur wissenschaftlicher Revolutionen.

LINDAU, V. (2019): Frei von Schuld. Die Macht der Vergebung. Talk-Episode 59, 13 February 2019, downloaded on 6 December 2020 from www.youtube.com/watch?v=7lrKrV2cnyM.

LEIBOLD, G. (1986): Körpertherapie.

LEWIN, K. (1951/2012): *Aus Feldtheorie in den Sozialwissenschaften [Field Theory in Social Science], selected theoretical writings*, translated by Lang, A. and Lohr, W.

LIEBL, F. (2001): Die Leute nicht für blöd halten. Depression und die Strategien ihrer Vermarktung, in Hegemann, C. (ed.): *Kapitalismus und Depression*, 3 volumes, III, 113–141.

LÖW, M. (2001): Raumsoziologie.

LOCKE, J. (1690/1997): An Essay Concerning Human Understanding.

LYOTARD, J.F. (1979/2012): *Das postmoderne Wissen*. Ein Bericht.

MARKOVÁ, I.S. / BERRIOS, G.E. (2019): Nature if the interactional field: psychopathological configurations, in Francesetti, G. / Griffero, T. (eds.): *Psychopathology and Atmospheres: Neither Inside Nor Outside*, 119–140.

MATT-WINDEL, S. (2017): Nähe – eine radikalhumanistische Perspektive auf Kontakt – eine Kernkompetenz der GT?, *Gestalttherapie*, 2/2017, 40–54.

MARX, K. (1852): Der achtzehnte Brumaire des Louis Napoleon, in Freiligrath, F. / Weydemeyer, J. (eds.): *Die Revolution, eine Zeitschrift in zwanglosen Heften*. 1 edition, I.

MATTHIES, F. (2013): Leibliche Kommunikation – Grundlagen des wechselseitigen Verstehens, *in Gestalttherapie: Forum für Gestaltperspektiven*, Vol. 27, No. 2, 77–95.

MATTHIES, F. (2015): Gibt es ein intersubjektives Feld, ein Zwischen und eine Kontaktgrenze?, *Gestalttherapie*, Vol. 29, No. 2, 89–99.

McCONVILLE, M. (2001): Let the Straw Man Speak Husserl's Phenomenology in Context, *Gestalt Review*, Vol. 5, No. 3, 195–204.

MEIER, A. (2017): Nach der Postmoderne, *in Postmoderne: Philosophie – Literatur*, downloaded on 12 January 2020 from www.literaturwissenschaft-online.uni-kiel.de.

MERLEAU-PONTY, M. (2002): Sinn und Nicht-Sinn.

METCALF, S. (2017): Die Idee, die die Welt verschlingt, *Freitag*, 21 December 2017, downloaded on 7 August 2020 from www.freitag.de.

MICHALITSCH, G. (2006): *Die neoliberale Domestizierung des Subjekts*. Von den Leidenschaften zum Kalkül.

MICHELS, C. (2015): Researching affective atmospheres, *in Geographica Helvetica*, Vol. 70, No. 4, 255–263.

MILLER, V. (2015): Resonance as a social phenomenon, *in Sociological Research Online*, Vol. 20, No. 2, 9, downloaded on 30 January 2020 from www.socresonline.org.uk/20/2/9.html.

MILLER, M.V. (2019): Beyond awareness, in Perls, F. / Robine, J.M. / Bowman, C. (eds.): *Psychopathology of Awareness*, 89–103.

MONBIOT, G. (2021): Trashing the planet and hiding the money isn't a perversion of capitalism. It is capitalism, *The Guardian*, 6 October 2021, downloaded on 11 April 2022 from www.theguardian.com.

MÜLLER, C. (2008): Neoliberale Körperreflexionen. Eine Analyse der Zurichtung des menschlichen Körpers im Neoliberalismus unter besonderer Berücksichtigung der emotionalen und körperlichen Panzerung, Magisterarbeit Universität Wien, Oktober 2008, downloaded on 30 August 2020 from https://core.ac.uk/download/pdf/11583243.pdf

NAGEL, T. (1974): What is it like to be a bat?, *in The Philosophical Review*. Cornell University, Ithaca, 83/1974, 435–450. downloaded on 20 June 2019 from web.archive.org.

NEATE, R. (2020a): Wealth of US billionaires rises by nearly a third during pandemic, *The Guardian*, 17 September 2020, downloaded on 6 November 2020 from www.theguardian.com.

NEATE, R. (2020b): Ten billionaires reap $400bn boost to wealth during pandemic, *The Guardian*, 19 September 2020, downloaded on 20 December 2020 from www. theguardian.com.

OBERHOFF, B. (2009): Übertragung und Gegenübertragung in der Supervision.

O'HAGAN, S. (2020): Health experts on the psychological cost of Covid-19, *The Guardian*, 7 June 2020, downloaded on 8 June 2020 from www.theguardian. com.

OLUSOGA, D. (2016): Black and British: A forgotten history.

PALZER, T. (2016): Spekulativer Realismus: Über eine neue Art, auf der Erde zu leben, Deutschlandfunk, 21 June 2016, downloaded on 30 March 2020 from www. deutschlandfunk.de.

PARLETT, M. (1997): The Unified Field in Practice, *Gestalt Review*, Vol. 1, No. 1, 16–33.

PARLETT, M. (2005): Contemporary Gestalt Therapy: Field Theory, in Woldt, A.L. / Toman, S.M. (eds.): *Gestalt Therapy: History, Theory, and Practice*, 41–63.

PENGELLY, M. (2016): 'Freedom or the idea of it': Does America need the existentialists, *The Guardian*, 9 April 2016, downloaded on 16 April 2020 from www.theguardian.com.

PERLS, F. (1947/1969): Ego, Hunger and Aggression.

PERLS, F. (1969/1992a): Gestalt Therapy Verbatim, [German edition] 1974.

PERLS, F. (1973): The Gestalt Approach & Eyewitness to Therapy.

PERLS, F. / Robine, J.M. / Bowman, C. (eds.). (2019): *Psychopathology of Awareness.*

PERLS, F. / HEFFERLINE, R.F. / GOODMAN, P. [PHG] (1951/2013): Gestalt Therapy: Excitement and Growth in the Human Personality.

PERLS, L. (1992): Living at the Boundary.

PETERSEN, L. (2020): Schöpferische Relationalität. Über das Dazwischen in der Gestalttherapie, *Gestalttherapie*, 2/2020, 25–38.

PETZOLD, H. (1977): Psychotherapie und Körperdynamik.

PETZOLD, H. (ed.). (1992): Die neuen Körpertherapien.

PETZOLD, H. (1996): Integrative Bewegungs- und Leibtherapie.

PHILIPPSON, P. (2009): The Emergent Self.

POLSTER, E. (1995): A Population of Selves. A Therapeutic Exploration of Personal Diversity.

POLSTER, M. / POLSTER, E. (1974): Gestalt Therapy Integrated. Contours of Theory & Practice.

POLUMBO, B. (2021): We're not really 'going back to normal' after the pandemic, 13 March 2021, downloaded on 16 September 2021 from www.washingtonexaminer. com/opinion.

RAPPE, G. (2018): Einführung in die moderne Phänomenologie.

REDECKER, E. von (2020): Es ist berauschend, die Probleme abzustreifen, in denen wir leben, Die Zeit online, 5 December 2020, downloaded on 10 December 2020 from www.zeit.de.

REICH, W. (1933/1971): Charakteranalyse.

REICH, R. (2020): To reverse inequality, we need to expose the myth of the 'free market', *The Guardian*, 9 December 2020, downloaded on 10 December 2020 from www.theguardian.com.

RESNICK, R. (2019): 'Narcissistic' buffoon or imperfect genius. The rehabilitation of a balanced view, in Perls, F. / Robine, J.-M. / Bowman, C. (eds.): *Psychopathology of Awareness*, 65–87.

RIEMANN, F. (1961/2011): Grundformen der Angst.

ROBINE, J.M. (1996): L'awareness, connaissance immediate et implicite du champ, *Cahiers de gestalt-thérapie*.

ROBINE, J.M. (2016): Comments on Griffero's lecture. Joint AAGT and EAGT gestalt conference, 22–25 September 2016 downloaded on 27 March 2017 from www.taorminaconference2016.com.

ROBINE, J.M. (2019): And Perls paid out for a codicil ..., in Perls, F. / Robine, J.M. / Bowman, C. (eds.): *Psychopathology of Awareness*, 187–195.

ROSA, H. (2019a): *Resonanz*. Eine Soziologie der Weltbeziehung.

ROSA, H. (2019b): Es geht um ein neues Gleichgewicht, Interview, in Stern, 8 August 2019, 32–33.

ROUBAL, J. (2019): Surrender to hope: The therapist in a depressed situation, in Francesetti, G. / Griffero, T. (eds.): *Psychopathology and Atmospheres: Neither Inside Nor Outside*, 69–100.

ROUBAL, J. / GECELE, M. / FRANCESETTI, G. (2016): Diagnose: Ein gestalttherapeutischer Ansatz, in Francesetti, G. / Gecele, M. / Roubal, J. (eds.): *Gestalttherapie in der klinischen Praxis*. Von der Psychopathologie zur Ästhetik des Kontakts, 79–104.

ROWAN, J. / JACOBS, M. (2002): The Therapist's Use of Self.

SALONIA, G. (2016): Sozialer Kontext und Psychotherapie, in Francesetti, G. / Gecele, M. / Roubal, J. (eds.): *Gestalttherapie in der klinischen Praxis*. Von der Psychopathologie zur Ästhetik des Kontakts, 185–195.

SAMADDER, R. (2019): Wellness or hellness? Nordic Cuddle therapy – Would you pay $65 to hug a stranger?, *The Guardian*, 11 June 2019, downloaded on 11 June 2019 from www.theguardian.com.

SARTRE, J.P. (1989): Ist der Existentialismus ein Humanismus? Three essays.

SARTRE, J.P. (1993): Das Sein und das Nichts.

SCHELER, M. (1913): Zur Phänomenologie und Theorie der Sympathiegefühle und von Liebe und Hass.

SCHELER, M. (1923): Wesen und Formen der Sympathie. Zur Phänomenologie der Sympathiegefühle.

SCHEURLE, H.J. (2013): Das Gehirn ist nicht einsam, Resonanzen zwischen Gehirn, Leib und Umwelt.

SCHEURLE, H.J. (2017): Resonanzen in der therapeutischen Beziehung, Psychosomatische Ansätze in der Psychotherapie, *Psychotherapie-Wissenschaft*, Vol. 7, No. 2, 39–48, downloaded on 9 February 2020 from www.psychotherapie-wissenschaft.info.

SCHMITZ, H. (1989): Leib und Gefühl.

SCHMITZ, H. (1999): Adolf Hitler in der Geschichte.

SCHMITZ, H. (2007): Der Leib, der Raum und die Gefühle.

SCHMITZ, H. (2011): Der Leib.

SCHNEE, M. (2018): Die Feldtheorie – ein Leuchtturm bei stürmischer See, *Gestalttherapie*, 1/2018, 29–50.

SCHREINER, P. (2015/2018): Unterwerfung als Freiheit. Leben im Neoliberalismus.

SCHREINER, P. (2019): "Freiheit ist das nicht", Interview mit Christian Baron, *Freitag*, No. 30, 25 July 2019, downloaded on 23 August 2020 from www.freitag.de.

SCHULZ, B. (2020): Häusliche Gewalt: Corona hält uns in der Hölle gefangen, *Zeit online*, 1 May 2020, downloaded on 14 June 2020 from www.zeit.de.

SERVAN-SCHREIBER, D. (2006): Die Neue Medizin der Emotionen. Stress, Angst, Depressionen: Gesund werden ohne Medikamente.

SCHWENKBECHER, J. (2019): Was einen guten Therapeuten ausmacht. Manche Therapeuten heilen die Leiden ihrer Patienten effektiver als ihre Kollegen, *Süddeutsche Zeitung*, 27 March 2019, downloaded on 17 May 2020 from https://www.sueddeutsche.de.

SIDDIQUE, K. (2020): The Political Economy of the Slave Trade – Capital Accumulation and the Rise of Britain, downloaded on 23 August 2020 from www.researchgate.net.

SÖNNICHSEN, B. (2020): Mein Helfer, der Pflege-Roboter, 10 March 2020, downloaded on 1 May 2020 from www.tagesschau.de.

SONNTAG, M. (1988): Die Seele als Politikum. Psychologie und die Produktion des Individuums.

SPAGNUOLO LOBB. (2013): The Now-for-Next in Psychotherapy. Gestalt Therapy Recounted in Post-Modern Society.

SPAGNUOLO LOBB. (2015): The body as a 'vehicle' of our being in the world. Somatic experience in gestalt therapy, *British Gestalt Journal*, Vol. 24, No. 2, November 2015, 21–31.

SPAGNUOLO LOBB. (2016): Grundlagen der Entwicklung der Gestalttherapie im Kontext der Gegenwart, in Francesetti, G. / Gecele, M. / Roubal, J. (eds.): *Gestalttherapie in der klinischen Praxis. Von der Psychopathologie zur Ästhetik des Kontakts*, 27–54.

SPAGNUOLO LOBB. (2017): Phenomenology and aesthetic recognition of the dance between psychotherapist and client: A clinical example, *British Gestalt Journal*, Vol. 26, No. 2, November 2017, 50–56.

SPAGNUOLO LOBB, M. (2018): Aesthetic Relational Knowledge of the Field: A Revised Concept of Awareness in gestalt, *Gestalt Review*, Vol. 22, No. 1, 50–68.

SPAGNUOLO LOBB, M. (2020): Dialogues on Psychotherapy at the Time of Corona Virus, *Introductory Presentation*, 15 May 2020.

SPAGNUOLO LOBB, M. / BLOOM, D. / ROUBAL, J. / ZELESKOV, J. et al. (2018): The aesthetic of otherness: Meeting at the boundary in a desensitized world. Taormina Conference, Proceedings.

STAEMMLER, F. (2001): Vorwort: 50 Jahre Gestalttherapie – Spekulationen zwischen den Zeiten, in Staemmler, F. (ed.): *Gestalttherapie im Umbruch. Von alten Begriffen zu neuen Ideen*, 9–31.

STAEMMLER, F. (2003): Ganzheitliches 'Gespräch', sprechender Leib, lebendige Sprache, *Edition Humanistische Psychologie*.

STAEMMLER, F. (2009): Das Geheimnis des Anders – Empathie in der Psychotherapie.

STANGL, W. (2020): Stichwort: Resonanzgesetz, *Online Lexikon für Psychologie und Pädagogik*, downloaded on 30 January 2020 from on www.lexikon.stangl.eu/16719/resonanzgesetz.

STARK, C. (2014): Neoliberalyse, Über die Ökonomisierung unseres Alltags.

STEPHENSON, F. (ed.). (1975): Gestalt therapy primer.

SIEFER, W. (2010): Die Zellen des Anstoßes, 17 December 2010, downloaded on 30 January 2020 from www.zeit.de/2010/51/N-Spiegelneuronen.

STORCH, M. / CANTIENI, B. / HÜTHER, G. / TSCHACHER, W. (2006): Embodiment – Die Wechselwirkung von Körper und Psyche verstehen und nutzen.

STRASSER, J. (2000): Triumph der Selbstdressur – Es zählt nur noch die profitable Verwertbarkeit. Über die Zurichtung des Menschen zu einem Element des Marktes, *Süddeutsche Zeitung*, 16–17 September 2000.

STRAUBHAAR, T. (2015): Neoliberalismus – Viele verstehen das Wort falsch, *Die Welt*, 14 April 2015, downloaded on 30 August 2020 from www.welt.de.

STRAUBHAAR, T. (2020): Kontrollierte Infizierung ist die beste Strategie gegen das Virus, *Die Welt*, 16 March 2020, downloaded on 30 August 2020 from www.welt.de.

TAYLOR, L. (2020): As our former lives dissolve into uncertainty, facts are something solid to cling to, *The Guardian*, 5 September 2020, downloaded on 6 November 2020 from www.theguardian.com.

THOMÄ, D. (2016): Soziologie mit der Stimmgabel, Zeit online, 30 June 2016, downloaded on 19 January 2020 from www.zeit.de.

VAN DE RIET, V. (2001): Gestalt Therapy and the Phenomenological Method, *Gestalt Review*, Vol. 5, No. 3, 184–194.

VERHAEGHE, P. (2014): Der neoliberale Charakter, *Freitag*, 24 October 2014, downloaded on 30 August 2020 from www.freitag.de.

VOLLAND, C. / ULRICH, D. / FISCHER, A. (1999/2004): Wer verdient Hilfe? Zum altersabhängigen Einfluss von Empfängermerkmalen auf die Prosozialität von Kindern, *Zeitschrift für Entwicklungspsychologie und Pädagogische Psychologie*, Vol. 36, 69–73. Published online on 1 April 2004.

WAGNER, W. (2019): Wie existenzialistisch ist die Gestalttherapie?, *Gestalttherapie*, 2/2019, 102–113.

WALCH, S. (2016): *Leibprozesse in der Gestalttherapie*, 1/2016, 109–121.

WATZLAWIK, P. / BEAVIN, J.H. / JACKSON, D.D. (1969): Menschliche Kommunikation.

WISEMAN, E. (2019): Are crystals the new blood diamonds?, *The Guardian*, 16 June 2019, downloaded on 29 April 2021 from www.theguardian.com.

WEGSCHEIDER, H. (2015): Das 'Zwischen' – ein intersubjektives Drittes, *in Gestalttherapie*, 1/2015, 3-24.0

WENGRAF, A. (2016): Gestalt – Erkenntnis – Theorie, *Gestalttherapie*, 1/2016, 2–22.

WENNINGER, G. (2000): Lexikon der Psychologie, *Feldtheorie Spektrum der Wissenschaft Verlagsgesellschaft*, downloaded on 30 March 2022 from www.spektrum.de/lexikon/psychologie/feldtheorie/4894.

WETZEL, D.J. (2016): Resonanz in der Soziologie Positionen, *Kritik und Forschungsdesiderata*, downloaded on 19 January 2020 from www.static1.squarespace.com.

WHEELER, G. (1991): Gestalt Reconsidered.

WHEELER, G. (2000): Beyond Individualism: Towards a New Understanding of Self, *Relationship, and Experience*.

WHO (World Health Organization). (2017): Depression and Other Common Mental Disorders, *Global Health Estimates*.

WIMMER, C. (2018): Die notwendige Kritik an einer Soziologie des Sockenstopfens, in Rezension von Peters, C.H. / Schulz, P. (eds.): *Resonanzen und Dissonanzen*, 18 January 2018, downloaded on 19 January 2020 from https://soziologieblog. hypotheses.org.

WOLLANTS, G. (2012): Gestalt Therapy. Therapy of the Situation.

YONTEF, G. (1993): Awareness, Dialogue & Process. Essays on Gestalt Therapy.

YONTEF, G. (2004): Zum Aspekt der Beziehung in Theorie und Praxis der Gestalttherapie, *Gestaltkritik 1-2004*, downloaded on 11 December 2016 from http://www.gestalt.de/yontef_dialog.html.

YONTEF, G. (2005): Gestalt therapy theory in change, in Woldt, A.L. / Toman S.M. (eds.): *Gestalt Therapy History, Theory and Practice*, 81–100.

ZAHAVI, D. (2007): Phänomenologie für Einsteiger.

ZEIT ONLINE. (2020): Wohlhabende verursachen mehr Kohlendioxid-Emissionen, 21 September 2020, downloaded on 6 June 2020 from www.zeit.de.

ZIELKE, O. (2017): Distanz und Distanzierung als therapeutische Kompetenz, in Conference booklet "Kernkompetenzen in der vielfältigen Praxis der Gestalttherapie", D-A-CH-Conference, Basel, 26–28 May 2017, 23.

ZILCHA-MANO, S. (2017): Is the alliance really therapeutic? Revisiting this question in light of recent methodological advances, *American Psychologist,* May 2017, downloaded on 14 January 2020 from www.researchgate.net.

ZINKER, J. (1977): Creative process in gestalt therapy.

ZULEEG, F. / EMMANOUILIDIS, J.A. / BORGES de CASTRO, R. (2021): Europe in the age of permacrisis, *European Business Review,* 11 March 2021, downloaded on 26 March 2022 from https://www.epc.eu/en/Publications.

Index